Anterior Resection of the Rectum

Single Surgical Procedures 6

A Colour Atlas of

Anterior Resection of the Rectum

Sir Hugh Lockhart-Mummery · Richard J. Heald · Ralph T. Hutchings

W DE G

Walter de Gruyter · Berlin · New York 1984

Sir Hugh Lockhart-Mummery KCVO, MD, MChir, FRCS; Consulting Surgeon, St. Thomas's Hospital, St. Mark's Hospital, London
Richard J. Heald MA, MChir, FRCS; Surgeon, Basingstoke Hospital, Hampshire
Ralph T. Hutchings, Photographer; Formerly Chief Medical Laboratory, Scientific Officer, Royal College of Surgeons of England

Original Publishers: Wolfe Medical Publications Ltd., · London
Exclusive co-publishers for the Federal Republic of Germany and Austria: Walter de Gruyter & Co., Genthiner Strasse 13, D-1000 Berlin 30. 1984.

Printed by Royal Smeets Offset b.v., Weert, Netherlands

Cover design: Rudolf Hübler

General Editor, Wolfe Surgical Atlases:
William F. Walker, DSc, ChM, FRCS (Eng.), FRCS (Edin.), FRS (Edin.)

CIP-Kurztitelaufnahme der Deutschen Bibliothek

Lockhart-Mummery, Hugh:
A colour atlas of anterior resection of the rectum /
Hugh Lockhart-Mummery; Richard J. Heald; Ralph T. Hutchings. -
Berlin; New York: de Gruyter, 1984.
(Single surgical procedures; 6)
ISBN 3-11-010017-7
ISBN 3-11-010016-9 (Subskr.-Pr.)
NE: Heald, Richard J.; Hutchings, Ralph, T.:; GT

Acknowledgements

We would like to record our thanks to Mr. Robert Lane, who produced the drawings of the technique of sutured anastomosis (Figures 36-42). We would also like to express our grateful thanks to our secretaries, Angela Dugdale, Rosemary Sexton and Jill Stevens, who have been of invaluable help in preparing the text; and to the many doctors and nurses who have helped in the production of this atlas.

Introduction

Anterior resection of the rectum is an abdominal operation in which the upper part of the rectum and its associated lymphatic field is removed, and continuity restored by anastomosis between the colon and the remaining ano-rectal segment. In a 'high' anterior resection, only the upper part of the rectum and the lower sigmoid colon are removed, and a rectal segment of 10 cm or so is left. In a 'low' anterior resection, the lower sigmoid and most of the rectum are removed and a short ano-rectal segment, perhaps only 4–5 cm long, is left for anastomosis. The 'low' operations are usually more difficult technically, and have a higher incidence of post-operative leakage. The operation is easier in a woman than in a man owing to the wider pelvis, and is always more difficult in fat people.

When doing any resection of the large bowel with anastomosis, one must ensure that both ends of remaining bowel being joined have a good blood supply and that they can come together without tension; and these principles must be firmly adhered to when doing an anterior resection. The blood supply of the distal ano-rectal segment is hardly ever in doubt, as there are rich vascular anastomoses between the middle and inferior haemorrhoidal vessels and other vessels of the pelvic floor. The length and blood supply of the colonic end, however, must always be carefully considered and checked. In most 'high' anterior resections the upper sigmoid colon can be brought down with good blood supply and without tension for anastomosis, but for 'low' anterior resections it may be necessary to mobilise the splenic flexure and to divide the left colic artery and vein. The descending colon can then be brought down low in the pelvis for anastomosis, relying on the marginal artery from the middle colic for blood supply.

The actual anastomosis may be carried out by suture, or by the use of the 'stapling gun'. Both these techniques are illustrated in this volume. It is usual to use a suture technique when the two ends of bowel to be joined are fairly accessible, but for very low anastomoses suturing can be extremely difficult and unsatisfactory, and a safer anastomosis can be carried out using the 'gun'.

The suture technique illustrated in this volume is a 2 layer method, using an outer interrupted seromuscular layer of 3.0 silk and an inner continuous all-coats layer of 3.0 Dexon or catgut. However, single-layer anastomoses using all-coats non-absorbable stitches are preferred by some surgeons and one of the authors (RJH) favours single-layer sero-muscular sutures that do not incorporate the mucosa. Despite such minor differences both the authors share a practical surgeon's preference for a manual anastomosis if this can be performed without undue difficulty. However, there is little doubt that the new stapling devices enable many surgeons to perform an anastomosis several centimetres lower than they would previously have attempted and thus perform more sphincter-conserving operations. A small reservoir of distal rectum can usually be left above the levators to provide discriminatory sensation and some reservoir function. Post operative continence is usually excellent if 2–3 cm or more can thus be spared above the anorectal ring and even colo-anal anastomosis provides acceptable continence in most patients.

The SPTU Russian gun was the first stapling device presented to Western surgeons. It can give good results if it is well maintained and the stapler washers and blades are re-loaded with obsessional care. It has, however, distinct dangers in the average busy operating suite with a variety of staff involved in its servicing and usage. For this reason most surgeons will choose one of the factory-packed disposable guns or cartridges marketed by the American Auto-Suture Company or by the Ethicon Company. The authors' preference is for the completely disposable Ethicon gun. This has the advantage of a particularly clean cut-off of the 'turned-in' bowel ends so that problems of withdrawal from the patient are very rare. There is a real danger that these 'guns' will lead to the performance of lower anterior resections without commensurate development of skilled low pelvic dissection technique. Such a trend would be disastrous and we have, therefore, tried in this volume to emphasise the details of pelvic dissection which are relevant to the proper excision of the tumour and its surrounding lymphatics. No aspect of rectal cancer surgery is more important than the avoidance of local recurrence.

Indications

The most frequent indication for this operation is for the treatment of a carcinoma arising in the upper rectum or recto-sigmoid junction. With increasing experience, and by the use of the stapling gun, it is now often possible to remove tumours of the mid-rectum by anterior resection and anastomosis, which in earlier years would have needed excision of the rectum and a permanent colostomy. In general, rectal tumours with the lower edge below 5 cm from the anal verge on sigmoidoscopy are not suitable for anterior resection; tumours with the lower edge between 5 and 10 cm may be suitable under favourable circumstances (a thin, preferably female, patient with a fairly small tumour); and those at 10 or more cm are usually suitable. Ideally, one should aim to remove 5 cm of bowel and associated mesorectum below the tumour, but a distal margin of 2–3 cm of bowel is sometimes acceptable, particularly if the mesorectum is adequately removed. If such a policy is followed the surgeon will find that between a half and three quarters of patients can be managed by anterior resection. After initial mobilisation of the rectum it becomes apparent whether or not the mesorectum and rectum can be divided comfortably 5 cm or more below the tumour. In such cases a high anterior resection with manual anastomosis is appropriate. If further mobilisation is required a deep pelvic dissection, division of the lateral ligaments, and probably a low stapled anastomosis will now be the choice of most surgeons.

In many cases the surgeon may not be able to tell whether an anterior resection will be the right operation for a particular patient, or even technically possible, until the abdomen has been explored and the growth mobilised. Whenever there is any such doubt, the patient should be warned before operation that an excision of the rectum and permanent colostomy may prove to be necessary, and consent for that obtained. Increasing familiarity with the deep pelvic dissection will lead to a higher proportion of sphincter-conserving operations, but cure of the malignant disease must always be the first consideration.

Other indications for anterior resection are for the removal of large benign (villous) tumours of the mid or upper rectum that cannot be fully dealt with by endoscopic methods per anum. Occasionally, diverticulitis or ischaemic disorders may lead to a stricture of the upper rectum suitable for anterior resection. Sometimes, malignant disease of the ovary or uterus may involve the rectum, and anterior resection may be necessary in clearing the pelvis of such a growth.

Contra-indications

Low rectal tumours are unsuitable, as are tumours found at operation to have extensive irremovable local pelvic dissemination; in such cases local recurrence is inevitable and would lead to obstruction and distressing symptoms.

A pre-operative biopsy that shows an anaplastic or very undifferentiated tumour of high malignancy is not now considered to be an absolute contra-indication to anterior resection. Nevertheless, such tumours disseminate more rapidly and widely within the pelvis and are more likely to permeate lymphatics and fat distal to the tumour. Thus a wide local clearance and a 5 cm distal margin are particularly needed in dealing with high grade tumours.

Pre-operative assessment

A general physical assessment of the patient's fitness for general anaesthesia and a major abdominal operation is obviously necessary in every case. Blood count, haemoglobin, urea and electrolytes should be checked, and arrangements made for transfusion if needed at operation, and before if the haemoglobin level is low. Chest x-ray and electrocardiogram are usually advisable. For large tumours, particularly those that feel fixed clinically, an excretion urogram (intravenous pyelogram) is advisable, as compression or displacement of one or both ureters may be demonstrated and the surgeon is duly warned. Excision appropriate to a malignant mass will often be more lengthy and difficult than the 'peeling-out' technique, which is satisfactory for an inflammatory one such as diverticulitis. Thus a recto-sigmoid lesion should have been accurately assessed pre-operatively by x-rays, endoscopy and, if possible, biopsy.

A double-contrast barium enema or a colonoscopy should be done on every patient unless there is gross obstruction. This is not to demonstrate the rectal tumour already diagnosed and assessed by finger and sigmoidoscope, but to demonstrate or exclude other tumours, benign or malignant, in the colon. In about 20% of patients adenomatous polyps are present elsewhere in the colon, and in about 3% of patients a second primary carcinoma is demonstrated. If the barium enema is done 3 or 4 days or more before the operation, the residual barium can be easily cleared from the bowel by the pre-operative preparatory routine.

Preparation

Ideally, the patient should come to operation with the large bowel nearly empty of faecal residue. This can be achieved partly by dietary measures (a low residue diet for 3–4 days pre-operatively, and clear fluids only for the last 24 hours) and partly and more effectively by purgation and/or washouts.

There are many methods of emptying the large bowel, of which the following are most used:

(1) Castor oil 30 ml orally 3 days pre-operatively, followed by the same dose 24 hours pre-operatively. No washouts or enemas are given. This is usually very effective, and not very unpleasant for the patient.

(2) Mannitol 10% – 1 litre is taken orally in 2 hours 2 days before operation, and repeated if necessary 24 hours pre-operatively. This produces rather more diarrhoea than castor oil but usually a clean empty bowel.

(3) Whole gut irrigation. A naso-gastric tube is passed and normal saline, with potassium chloride 1 g per litre added, is given through it at the rate of 2 litres per hour. 10 mg of Maxolon (metoclopramide) is given i.m. at the start and the saline infusion continued until the rectal evacuant is clear. This method is unpleasant for the patient, who may need to spend some hours on a commode, but produces a very clean empty bowel.

Irrigation and washouts of the colon may also be used, but are more unpleasant for the patient, require more nursing procedures than the purgation regimens, and seem to be no more effective. No aperient should be given within 18 hours of surgery for fear of producing an active colon laden with semi-liquid stool.

In spite of preparation by one of the above methods, patients with somewhat obstructive lesions may be found at laparotomy to have an unacceptably loaded colon. In these circumstances the bowel may be washed through in the operating room, from the terminal ileum to the point of division of the left colon in the manner described by Dudley et al (Brit. J. Surg. 1980 *67* 80–81).

It is not our practice now to give routine pre-operative antibiotics or sulphonamides to reduce bowel flora. We now prefer per-operative systemic protection of the patient by antibacterials. At the start of the operation, metronidazole 1 g is given intravenously, and then 0.5 g i.v. is given 12 hourly from the evening of the operation for 48 hours. Some surgeons also include a broad spectrum anti-aerobic agent and others now prefer a single 'third generation' cephalosporin to cover both aerobes and anaerobes.

In the anaesthetic room, an intravenous drip is put in place and a balloon catheter is passed into the bladder and connected to a draining-bag.

1

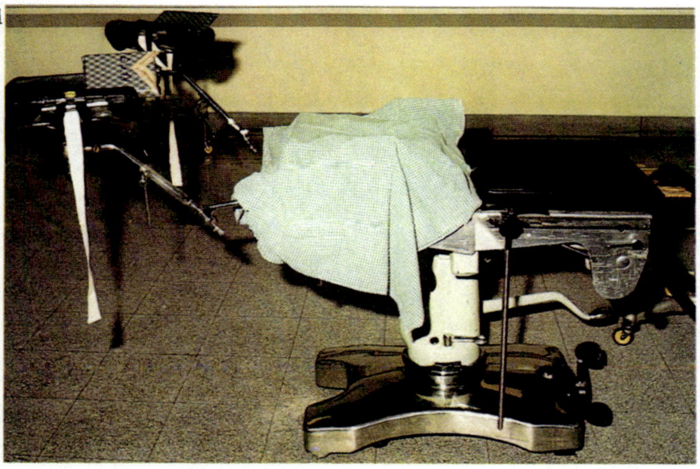

2

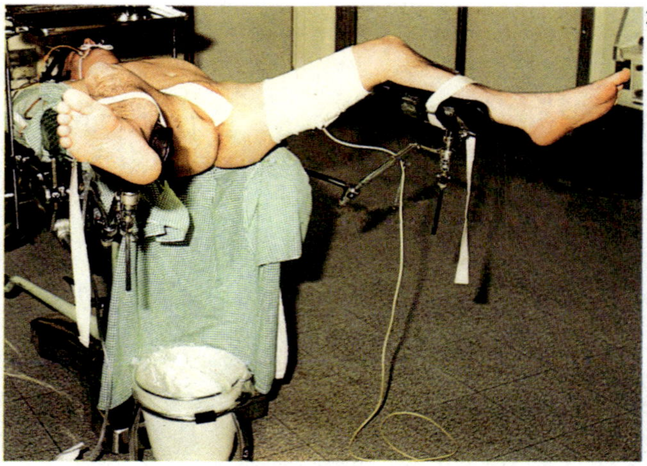

Patients for anterior resection should be operated on in the lithotomy-Trendelenburg position (Lloyd-Davies 1939), which allows unimpeded access both to the abdomen and the anus and perineum.

1 The table set up The upper and lower leafs are removed and the special leg pieces are in position. A padded pelvic support is in position covered with a waterproof material.

2 The patient on the table Note particularly that the legs are strapped into the leg supports and that the anus and perineum are well over the end of the pelvic support, on which the most prominent part of the sacrum should rest. The diathermy pad is in position on one thigh and the catheter (and penis and scrotum in a male patient) is held with adhesive plaster over the right groin.

3

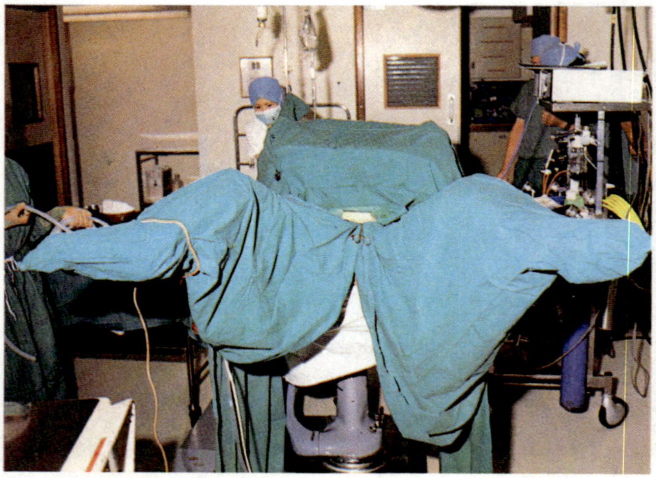

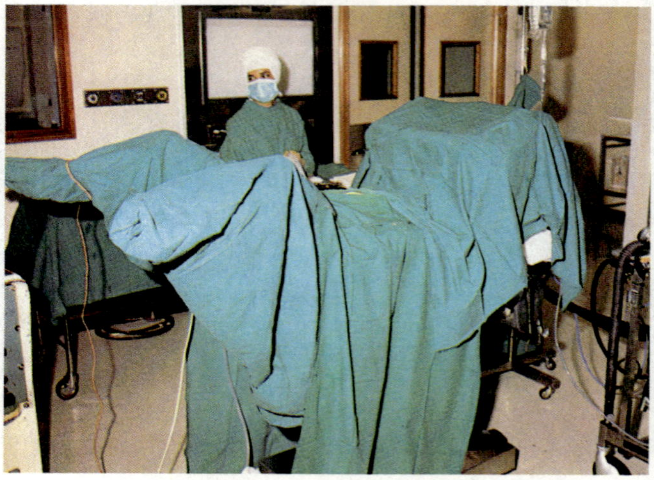

4

3 and 4 The towelling of the patient in this position Special large triangular leggings are very useful in covering the legs, yet allowing good access to the anus. The abdominal towelling should allow for a full length abdominal incision, and an instrument tray over the patient's chest is useful.

5

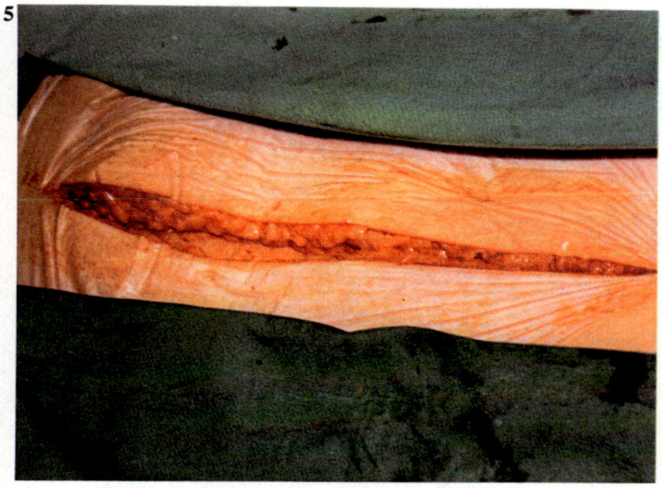

6

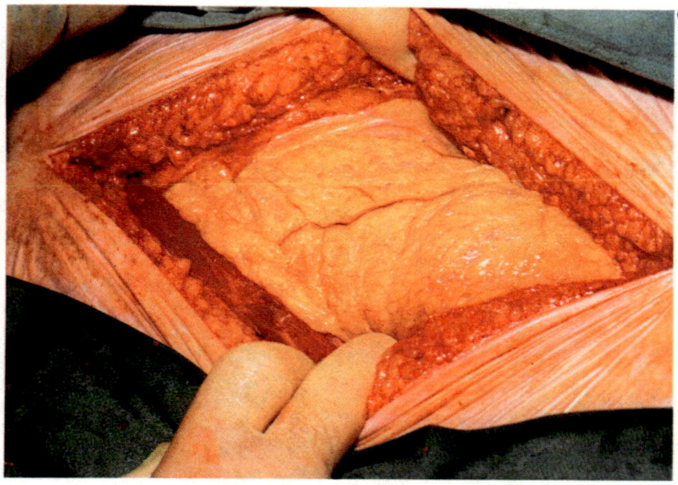

5 A long left paramedian incision allows excellent access It should start at the pubis and be carried at least three inches above the umbilicus. In cases in which the splenic flexure is mobilised there should be no hesitation in extending it to the costal margin.

6 Abdomen open The first step is to explore the liver manually for possible secondaries. The peritoneal cavity and omentum are seen and felt for seedling deposits. The gall-bladder, stomach, oesophageal hiatus and small bowel are felt. The whole colon is then examined, although the pre-operative barium enema or colonoscopy should have screened for any disease other than the tumour in the rectum.

7 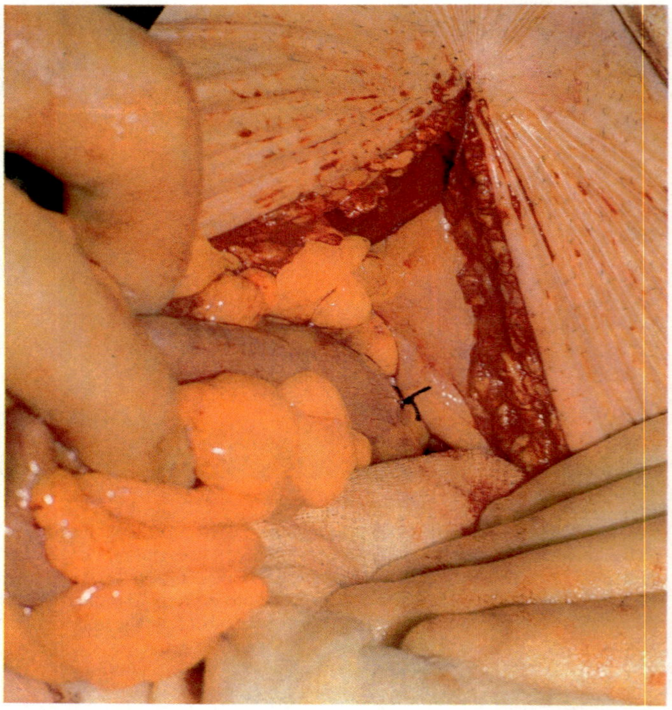

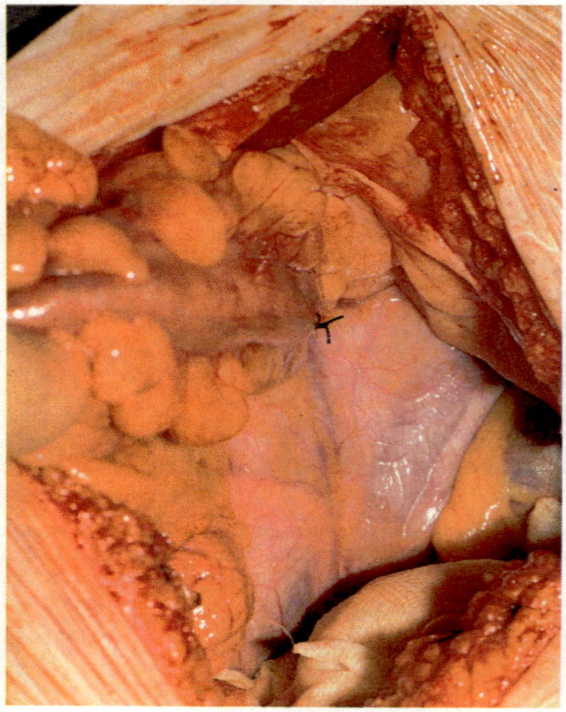 8

7 The table is tilted about 15–20° head-down (too steep a tilt makes the operation more difficult) and the pelvis is then inspected and palpated. The site, size and mobility of the tumour is assessed, the mesorectum and para-aortic region felt for enlarged nodes, and the presence of any local peritoneal spread noted. If the tumour is small and not very obvious, its lower border should be marked with a black stitch in the seromuscular layer.

A large, moist gauze pack is now being used to cover the small bowel and caecum and pack them upwards.

8 The small intestine has now been packed away and the pelvis is clear. The small tumour (at the recto-sigmoid junction in this case) is marked.

9

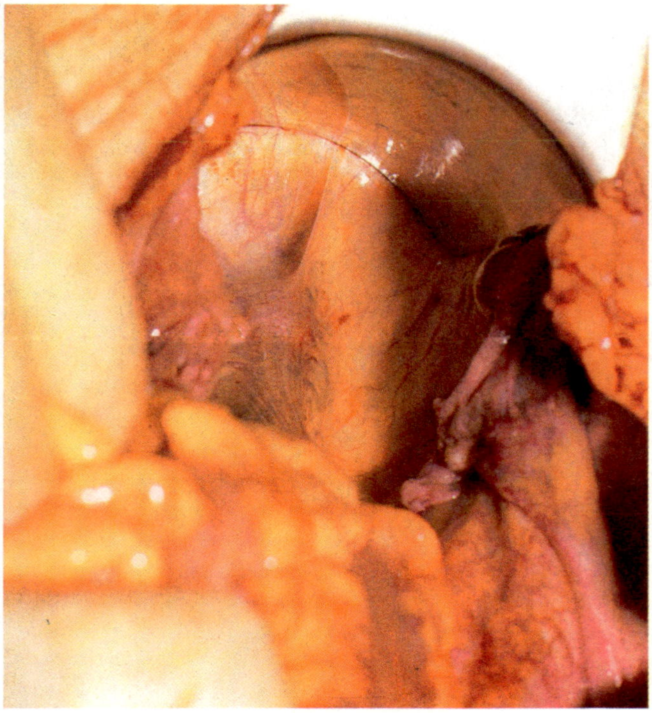

10

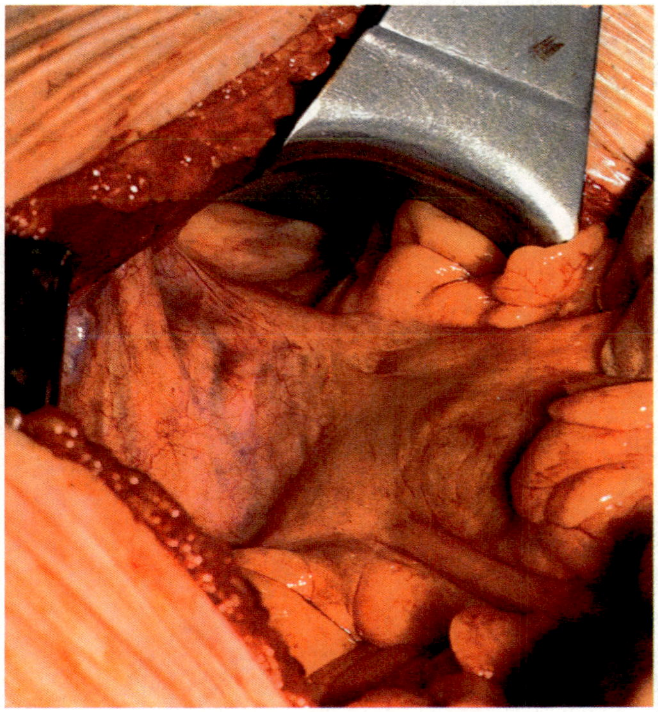

9 Similar view in another case. In this female patient the rectal tumour is visible just above the peritoneal reflection.

10 A large self-retaining retractor is inserted to hold the wound edges apart. The assistant holds the sigmoid colon upwards and to the right.

11

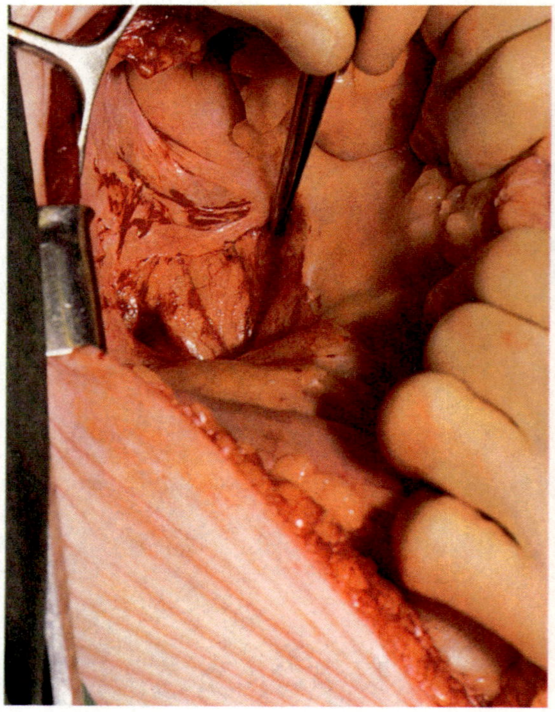

11 The surgeon starts the operation by dividing the congenital adhesions on the left side of the sigmoid colon, exposing the retroperitoneal tissues and finding the left ureter and ovarian or testicular vessels.

12

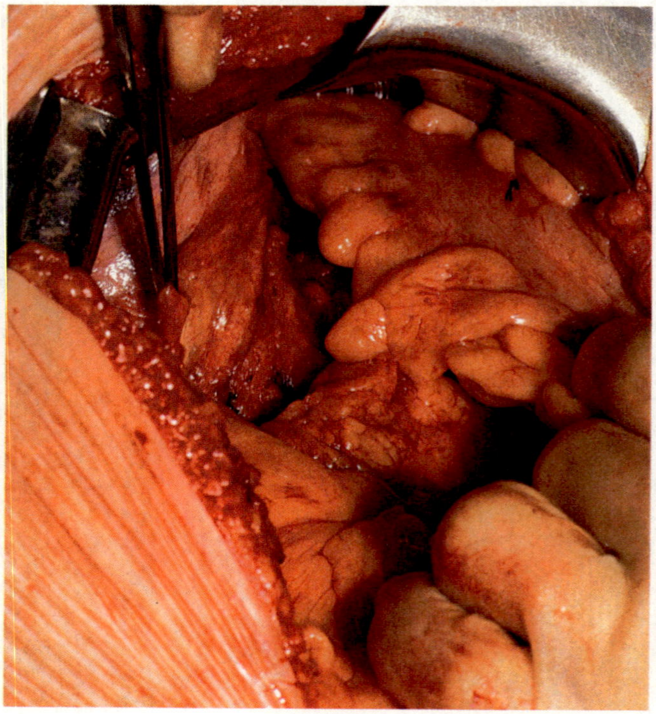

12 This peritoneal cut is extended downwards into the pelvis, exposing and preserving the ureter, which is gently pushed laterally.

13

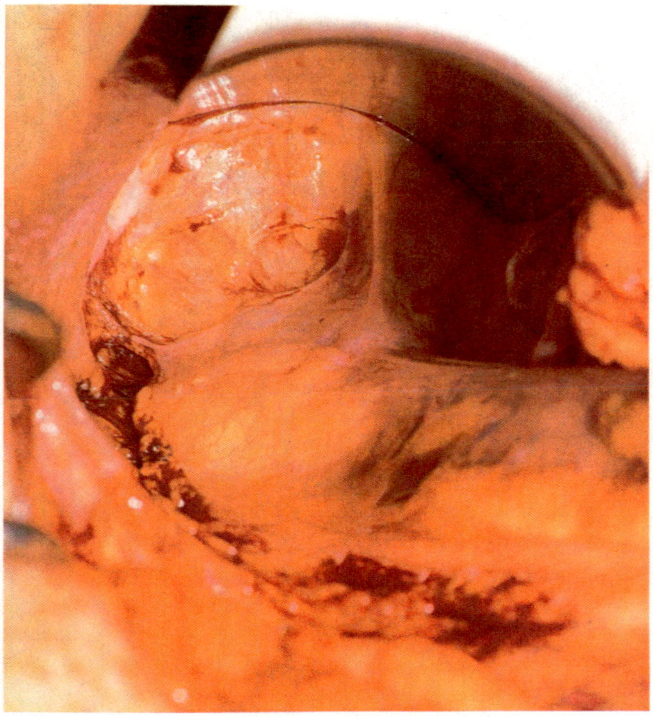

14

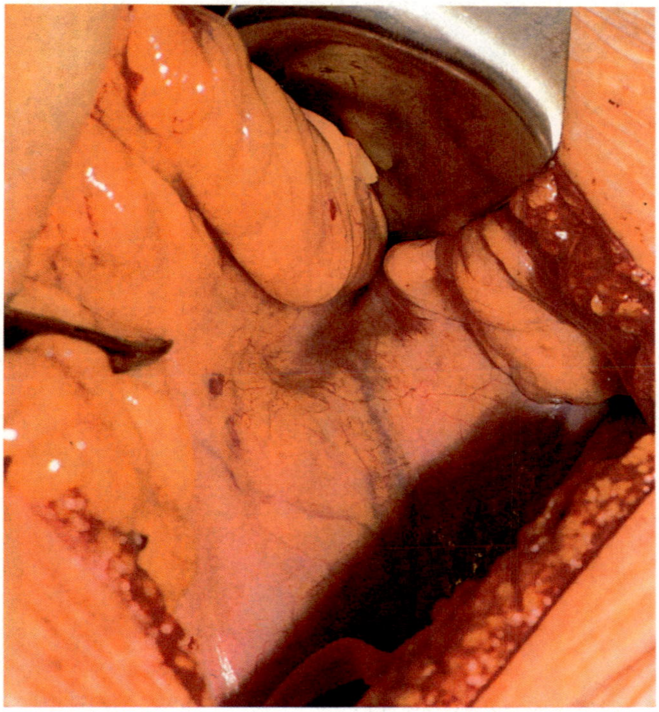

13 Another case. The peritoneal cut has here been extended to the bottom of the pelvis and taken across the front of the rectum below the tumour.

14 The sigmoid is now held to the left and the right peritoneal leaf opened, leaving sufficient peritoneum for suturing without tension at the end of the operation.

15

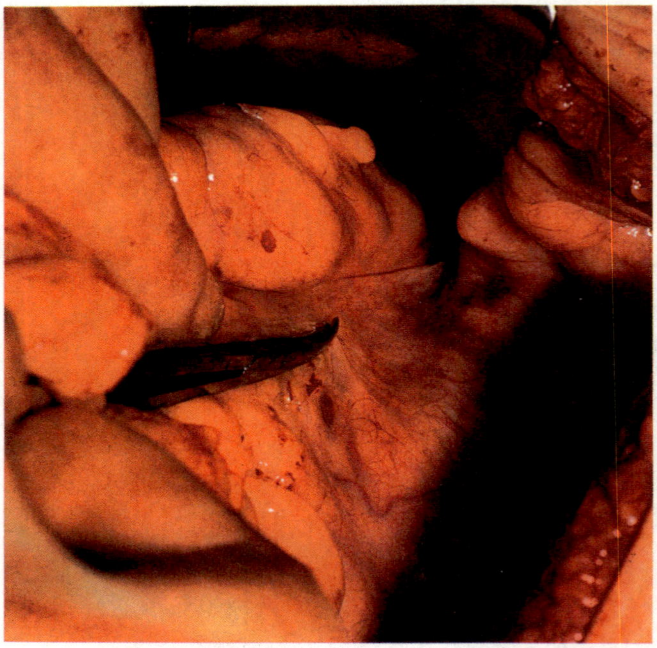

16

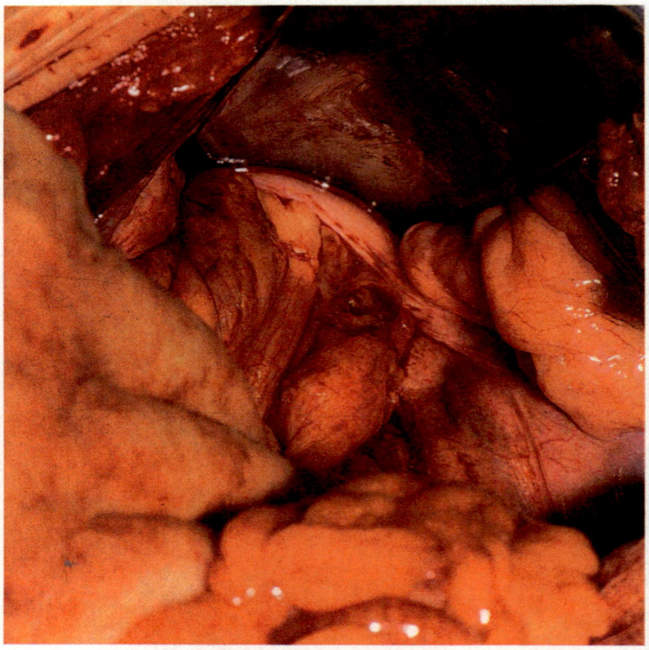

15 The peritoneal cut is carried deeper into the pelvis. The right ureter may be seen, but it is usually well out of the way.

16 The peritoneal cuts are joined across the front of the rectum. Note the value of a deep and wide retractor anteriorly when working deep in the pelvis.

17

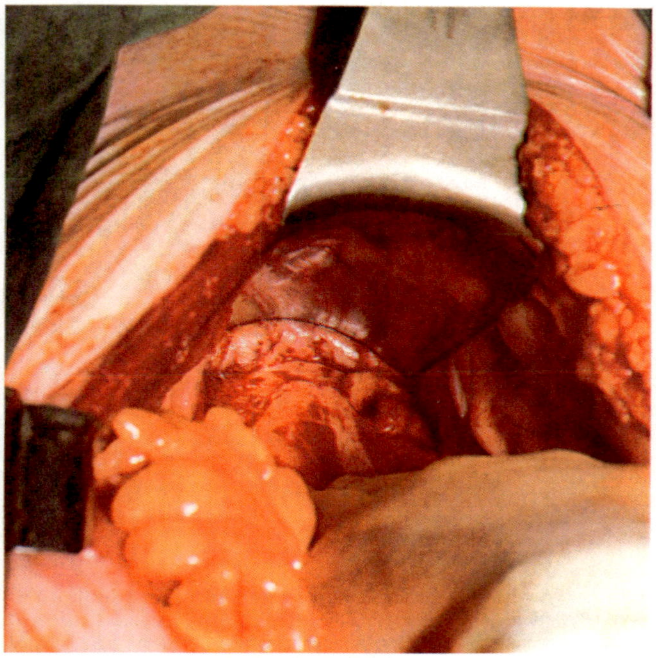

17 Another case, with a lower tumour. The peritoneal cuts have been joined anteriorly, and the posterior wall of the seminal vesicles is exposed.

18

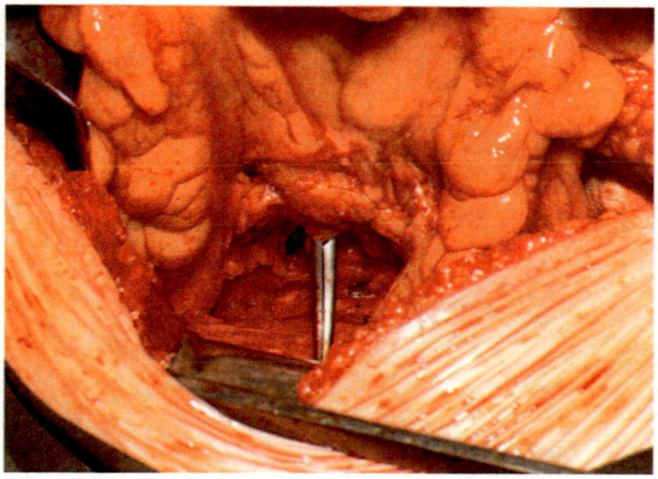

18 Attention is now turned to the main vessels and the ligation of the vascular and lymphatic pedicle.

By gentle finger or gauze dissection the main superior haemorrhoidal vessels are freed from the common iliac vein, aortic bifurcation and sympathetic tissue of the posterior abdominal wall, until a finger or haemostat can be passed beneath them.

19 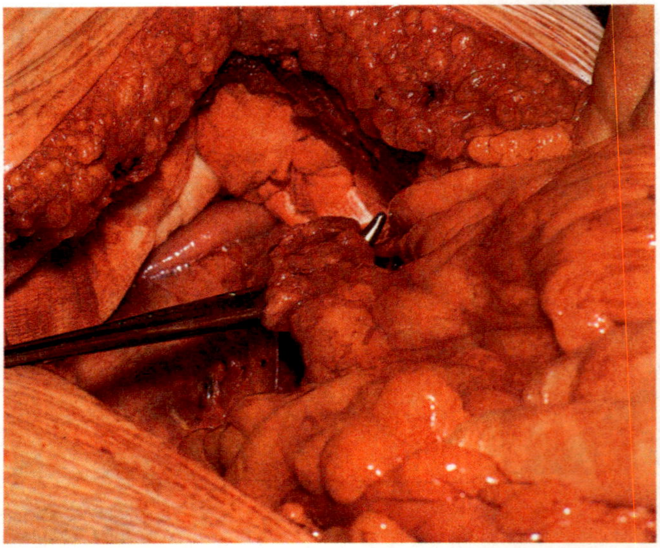

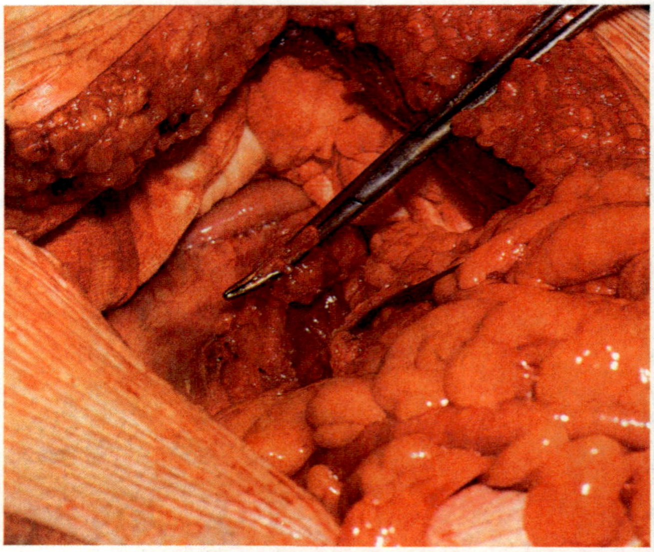 20

19 The assistant now retracts the upper end of the wound, the peritoneal cut is extended upwards and the main vessels defined and cleaned about level with the aortic bifurcation. (*The camera is looking towards the head of the table in this and the next two figures*)

20 The superior haemorrhoidal vessels have been clamped and divided. This can usually be done below the origin of the left colic and main sigmoid arteries. If a 'high tie' is considered necessary, the artery may be tied near the origin from the aorta and the vein separately at the same level.

21

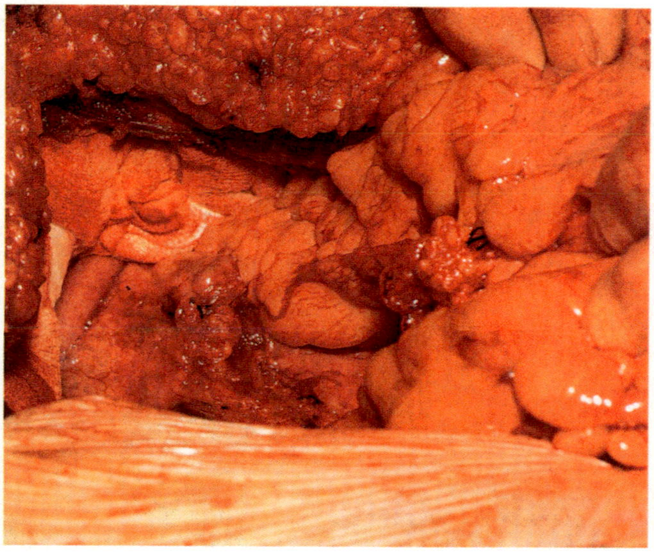

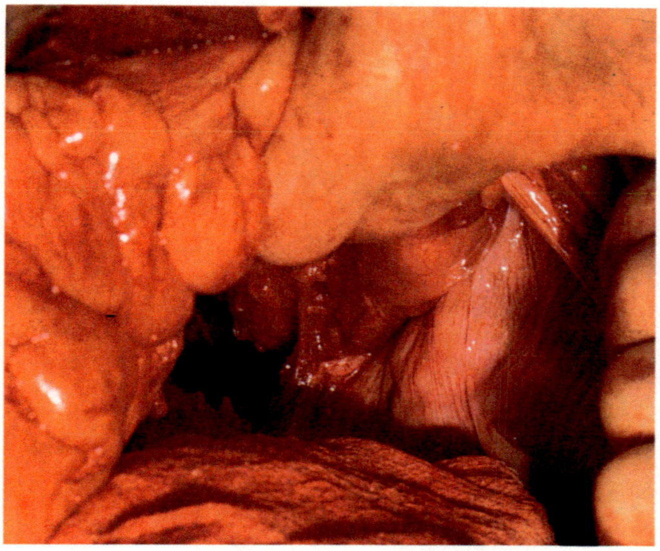

22

21 Both ends have been safely ligated with silk. The lower sigmoid colon and its mesentery can now be lifted further forward and freed from the posterior abdominal wall by gentle scissor dissection.

The camera is now again directed into the pelvis.

22 The rectum is freed further posteriorly by holding it forward and gently dividing the fascial strands that hold it in contact with the posterior wall. The left common iliac vein lies above the sacral promontory but, below this, in front of and below the sacral promontory, there is no vital structure and the plane usually opens up easily.

The dissection should be kept strictly in the midline until the plane is defined and is then extended to the postero-lateral aspects so that the rectum is gradually mobilised forward. The sympathetic trunks on each side, which run over the great vessels and then down on to the pelvic side walls, can usually be seen and should be preserved.

23 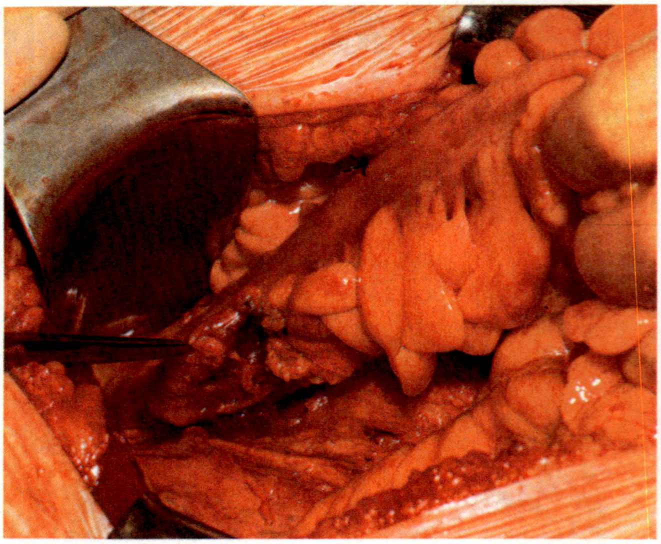

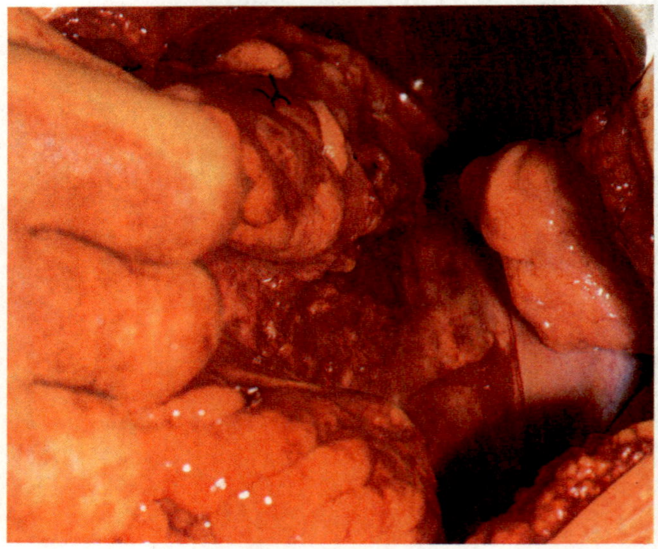 24

23 In a 'high' anterior resection, little more mobilising of the rectum may be necessary. In such a case, the peritoneal cut on the left side is now taken to the side of the rectum at a sufficient distance below the tumour (ideally 5 cm), clearing the rectum of fat and ligating or coagulating small vessels.

24 The peritoneal cut on the right side is now taken to the side of the rectum at the same level.

25

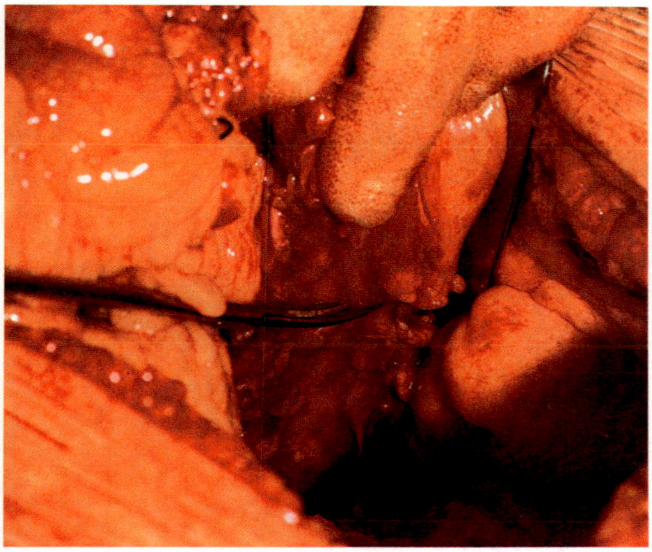

26

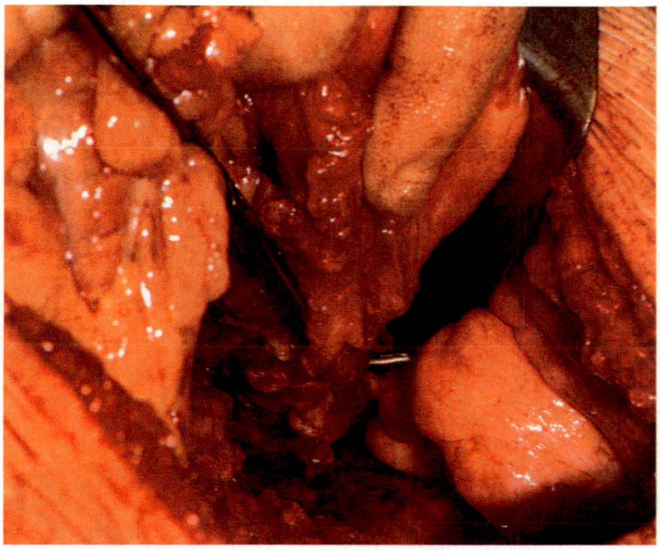

25 The rectum is held forward and the posterior fascia surrounding the vessels in the mesorectum is divided at the same level.

26 This exposes the superior haemorrhoidal vessels, which can be isolated from the bowel, picked up with curved haemostats, divided and ligated.

27 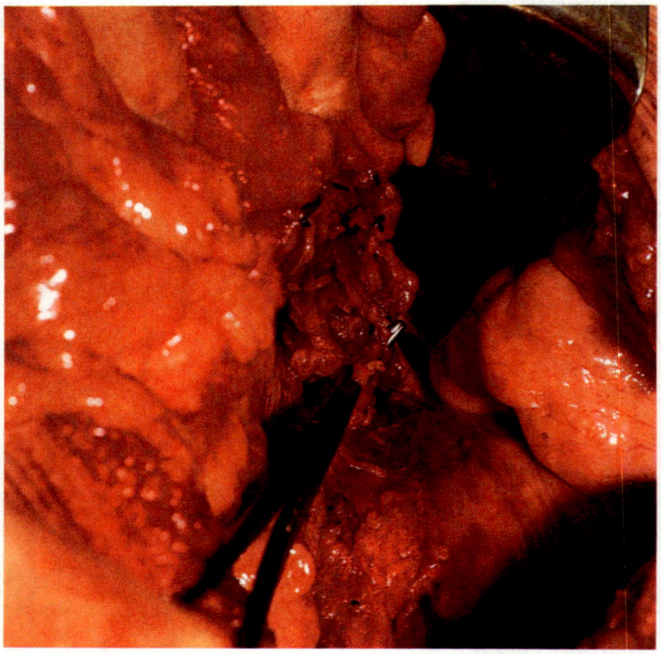

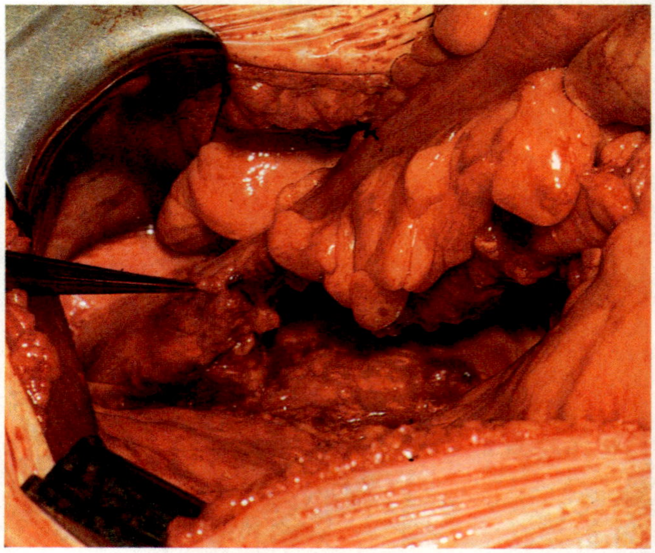 28

27 There may be more than one leash of vessels to divide, but after dealing with them all the dorsal aspect of the rectum is exposed and clear.

9

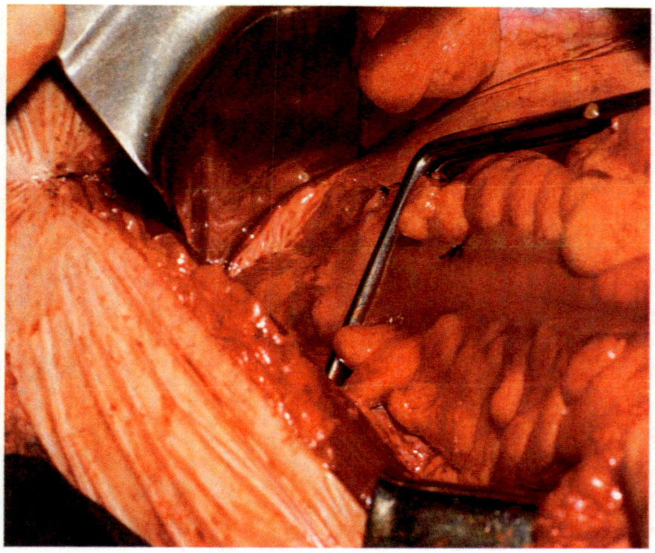

29 A firm right-angled occlusion clamp is now applied right across the rectum, just above the cleared segment, so that the rectum can be divided below the clamp, through the prepared area.

30

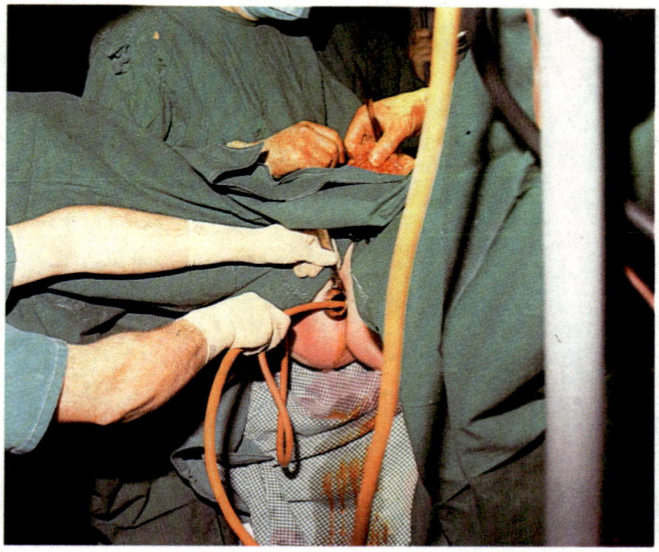

30 When the clamp has been applied, the rectum should be washed out from below by an assistant. A proctoscope is passed and the rectum irrigated from a reservoir through wide-bore tubing, so that a good flow is obtained. Distilled water, a mild antiseptic solution, or 1 in 1000 perchloride of mercury may be used, and irrigation continued until the rectum is clean. The rectum is then mopped dry with gauze before removing the proctoscope.

The main aims of the washout are to remove or destroy any malignant cells in the bowel lumen that might implant on the suture line, as well as to attain a clean and empty bowel for anastomosis.

31

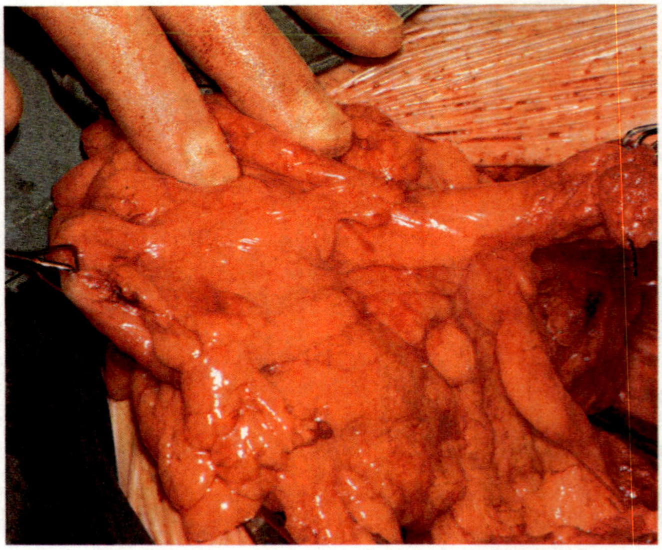

32

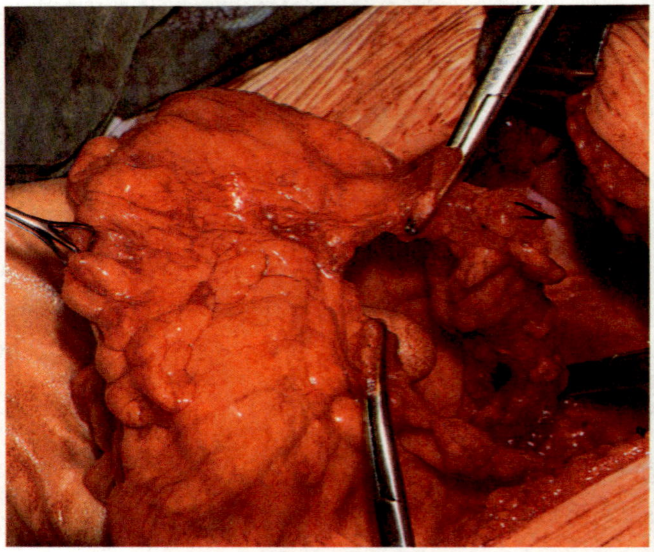

31 While the washout proceeds, the surgeon now turns his attention to the proximal colon. He must decide whether the sigmoid colon is sufficiently long and mobile to come down for anastomosis to the remaining rectum without any tension, or whether the splenic flexure should be mobilised to obtain more length of bowel. For most 'high' resections, the sigmoid colon can be used. (see later for use of more proximal bowel).

The sigmoid colon and its mesocolon are held over to the left. Unless there is much fat the actual vessels can usually be seen. The exact point on the bowel at which the surgeon wishes to divide it is marked with Babcock or similar light forceps.

32 The mesocolon is carefully divided, picking up and tying any vessels. When nearing the bowel, it is comforting to divide a small vessel without prior clamping to make sure that the proximal end bleeds freely.

3

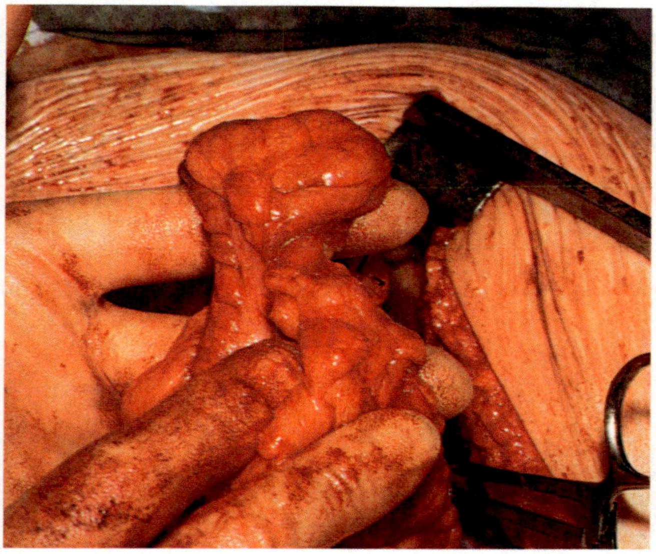

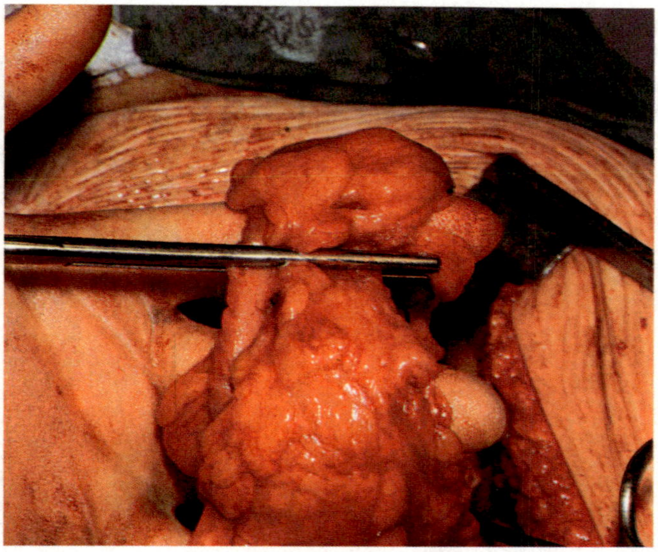

34

33 The mesentery has been divided and a small segment of the colon wall has been cleaned and bared.

34 An occlusion clamp is applied across the colon in the bared segment.

35

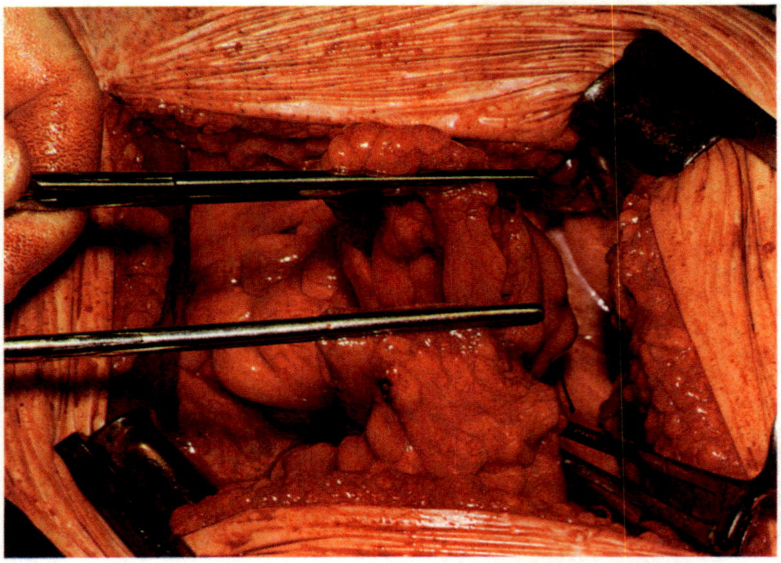

35 A second clamp is applied immediately distal to the first, and the bowel divided between them.

36

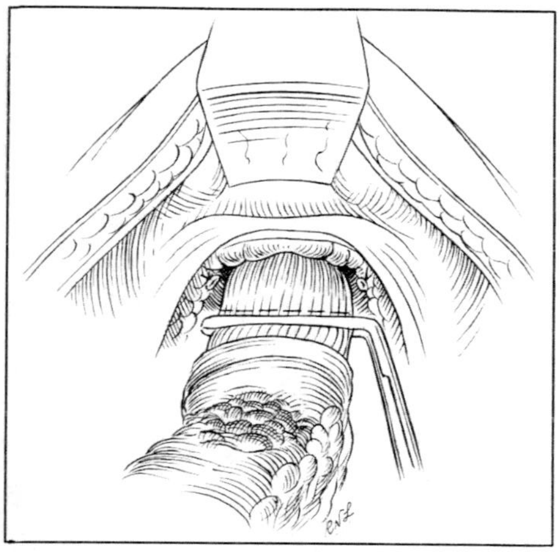

37

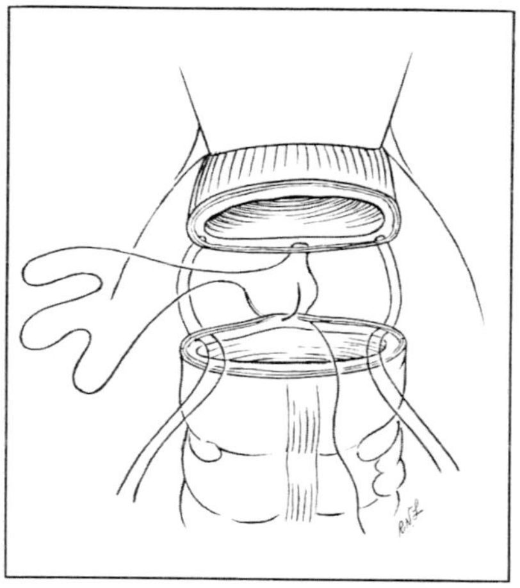

38

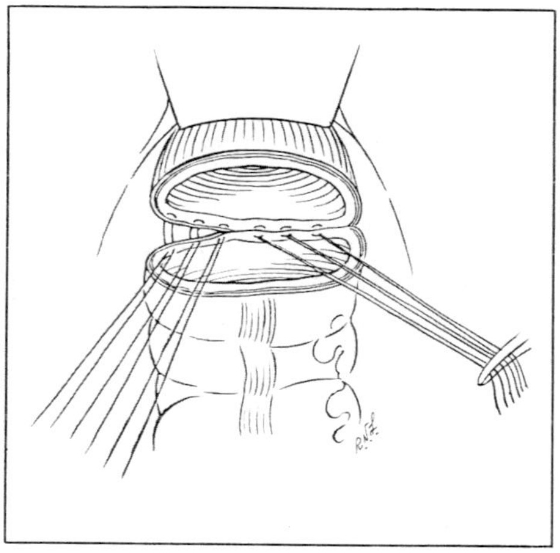

The line drawings show the technique for the final stages of the operation.

36 The rectum is divided below the clamp.

37 Interrupted silk stitches are then placed in the posterior walls of both rectum and colon, which are still widely separated. 5 or 7 stitches are usually needed.

38 The colon is then pushed down into the pelvis and the stitches tied, thus joining the two ends of the bowel.

39

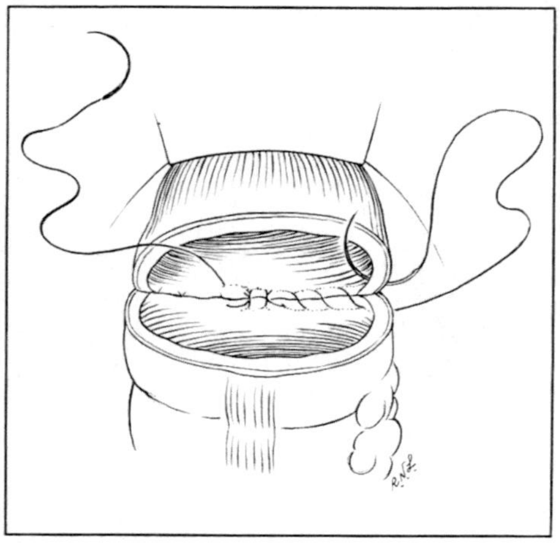

40

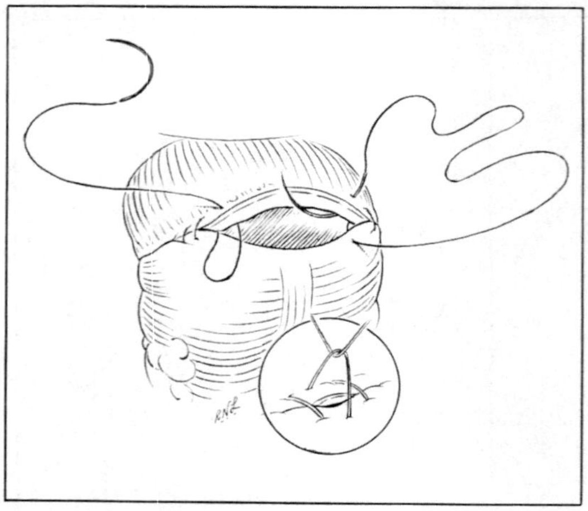

41

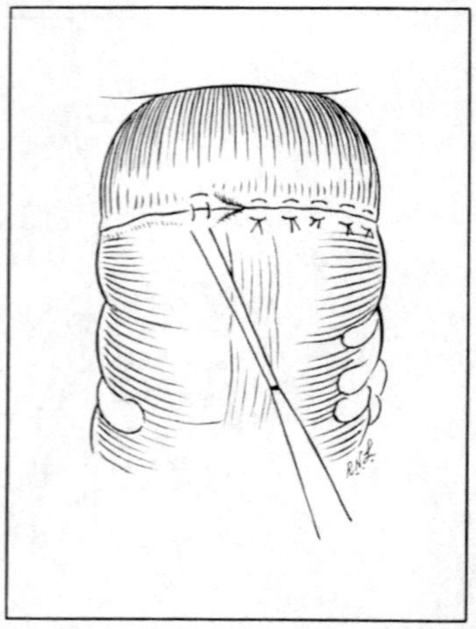

39 A continuous all-coats suture is then inserted; two separate lengths of atraumatic catgut or Dexon are used, each starting in the centre of the back wall and going round each side.

40 These sutures are then continued on the anterior wall as Connell inverting sutures, and finish, tied together, in the middle of the anterior wall.

41 An anterior row of interrupted silk sutures is then used to bury the all-coats suture.

42

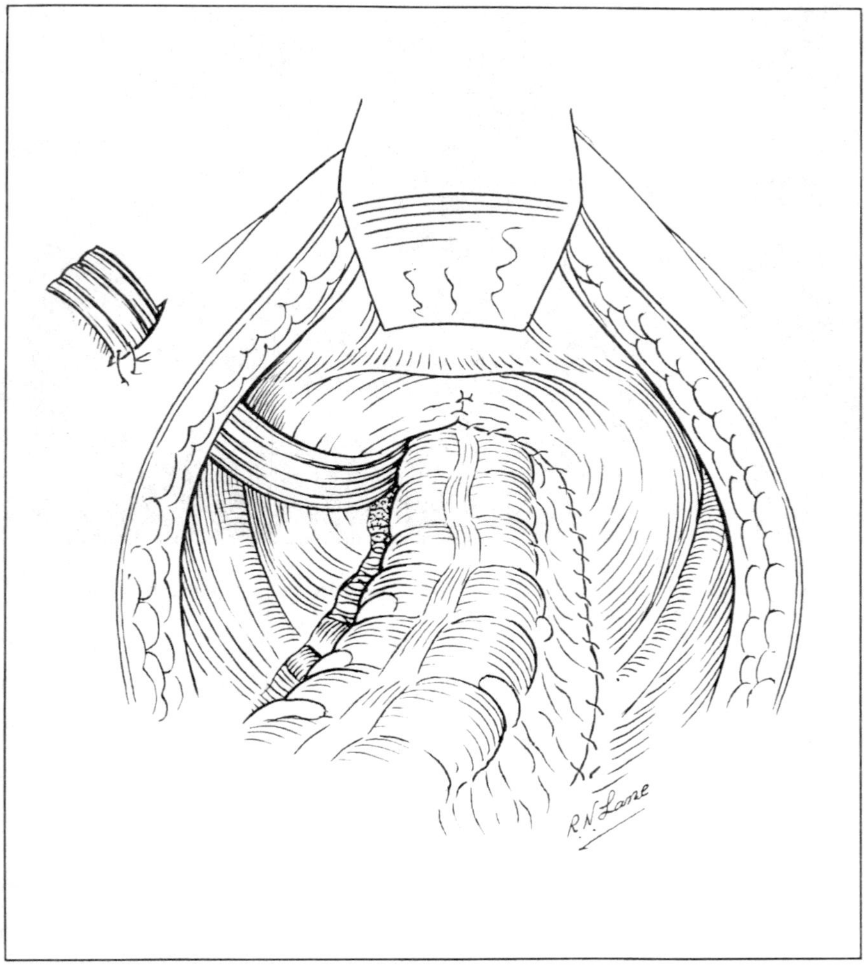

42 The front and right side of the pelvic floor is closed, sewing the right leaf of peritoneum to the mesocolon (being very careful not to damage the vascular supply to the bowel). A drain is placed in the pelvis behind the anastomosis on the left side and brought out through a stab incision in the left iliac fossa.

43

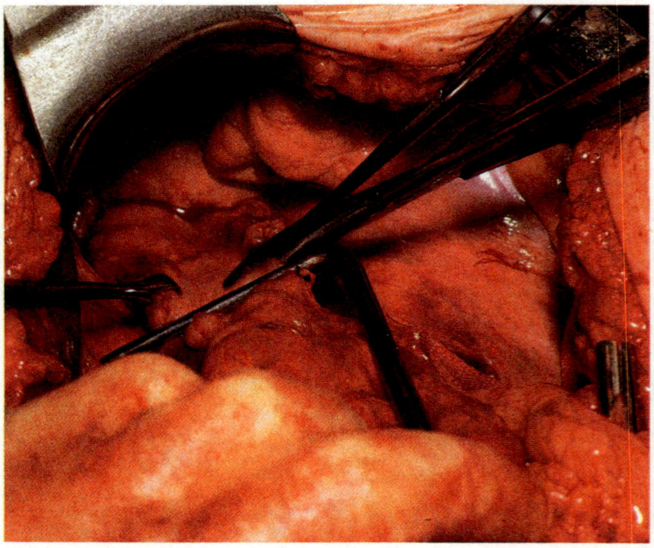

43 The rectum is being divided below the clamp with curved scissors. Long Babcock's forceps hold the rectum.

44

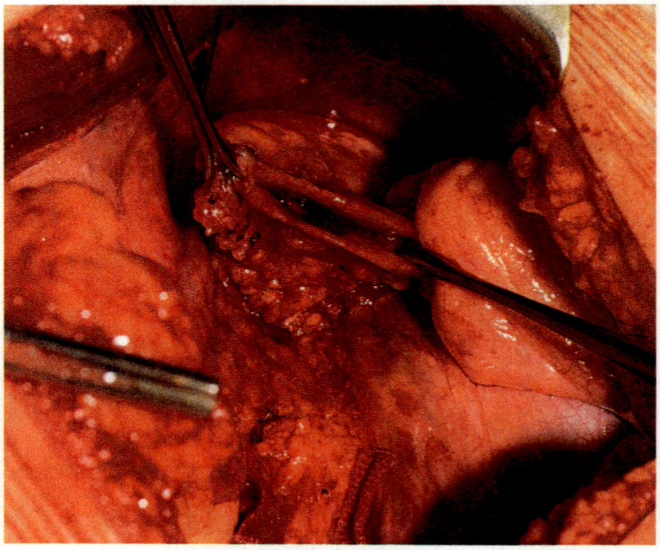

44 The rectum has been fully divided and the specimen removed. The rectum is held with Babcock's forceps.

45

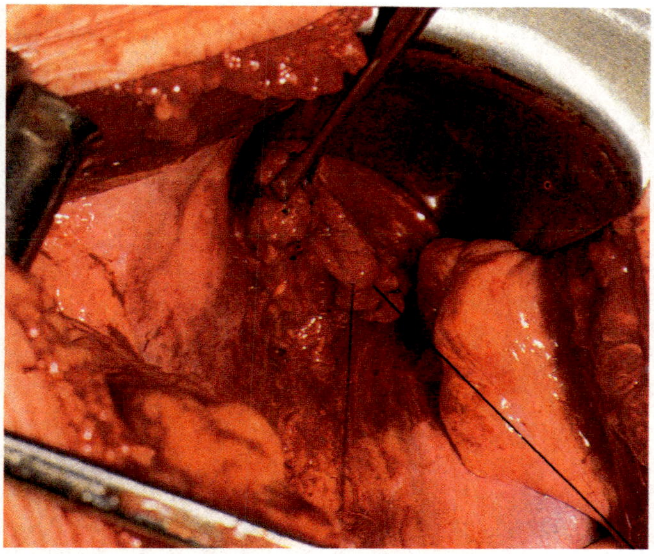

45 The first dorsal seromuscular stitch has been inserted. It is best to put in the two end ones first, then one in the middle, and then the remaining two or four between them. In this way any disparity in the size of the two ends can be accommodated.

46

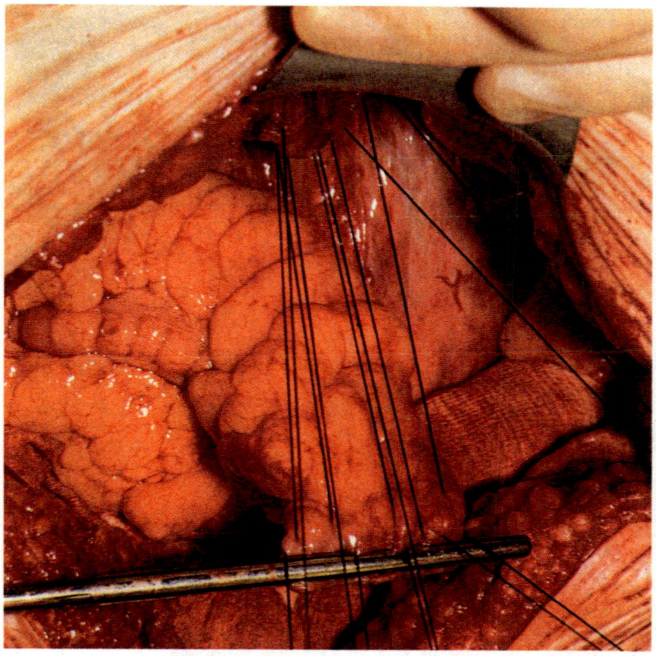

46 Five posterior seromuscular stitches have now been placed.

47

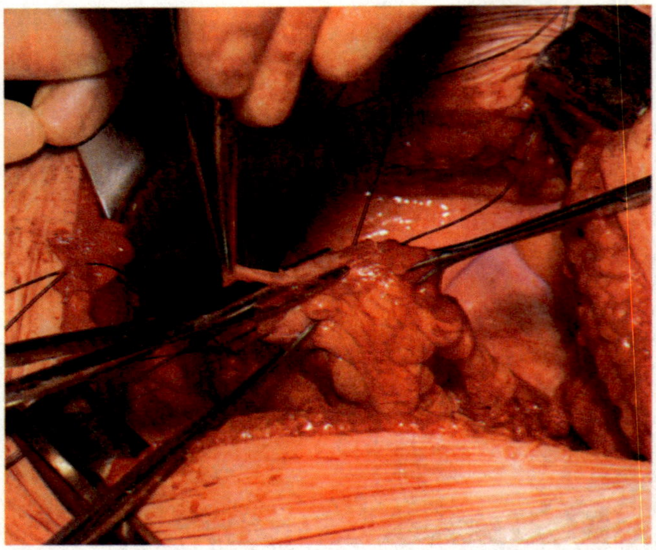

47 The clamp has now been removed from the upper end, which is held with Babcock's forceps. The thin sliver of crushed bowel is cut off with scissors. The sucker should be ready at this stage to deal immediately with faecal contamination.

48

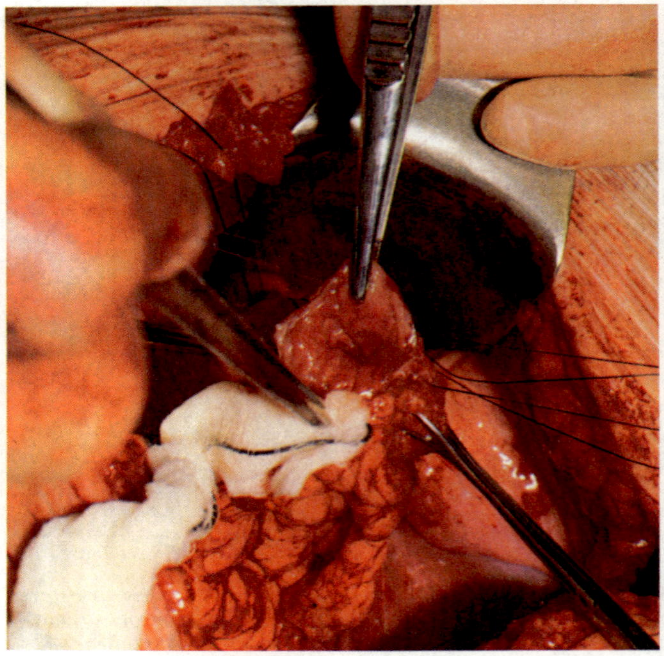

48 The proximal colon is mopped clean with a mild antiseptic solution.

49

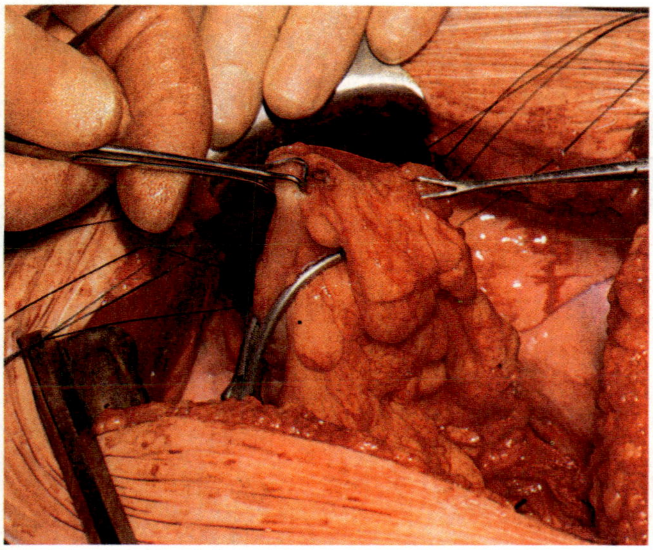

50

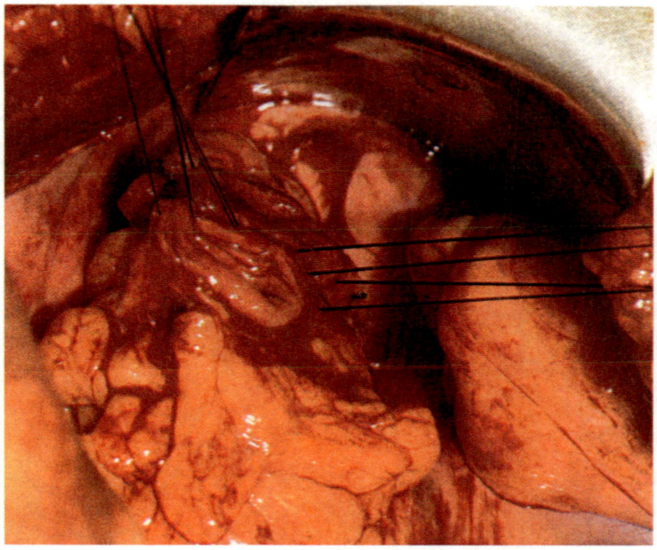

49 A light occlusion clamp across the bowel prevents any soiling during the anastomosis. A De Bakey vascular clamp is very suitable as there is no long handle to get in the way.

50 The colon has been 'railroaded' down the sutures and the two ends are now joined.

51

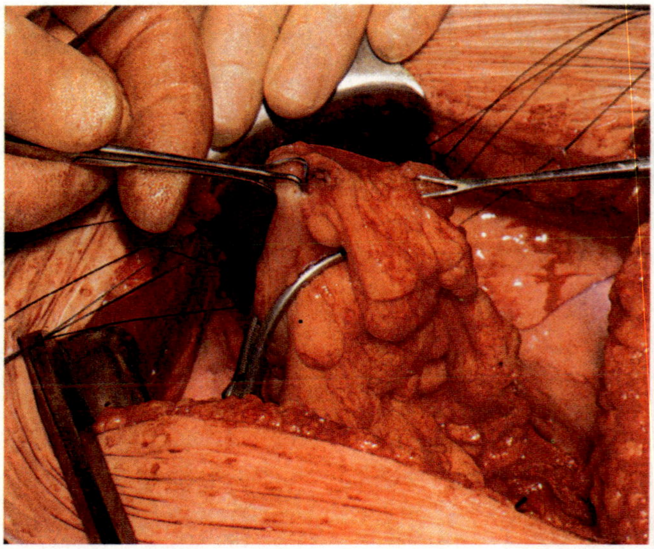

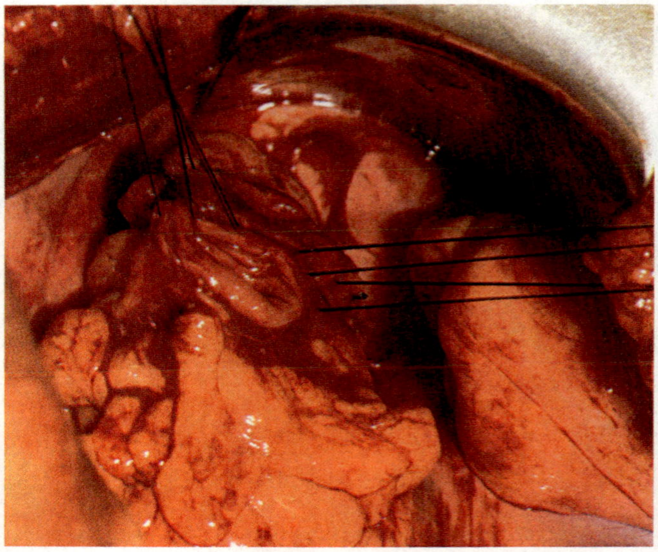

52

51 All sutures have now been tied. The central and end ones are held, and the others cut.

52 The first all-coats Dexon or catgut suture has been inserted in the middle of the posterior wall and tied. The shorter end is held up and to the right, and stitching proceeds from centre to left along the posterior wall. The central silk suture can now be cut short.

53

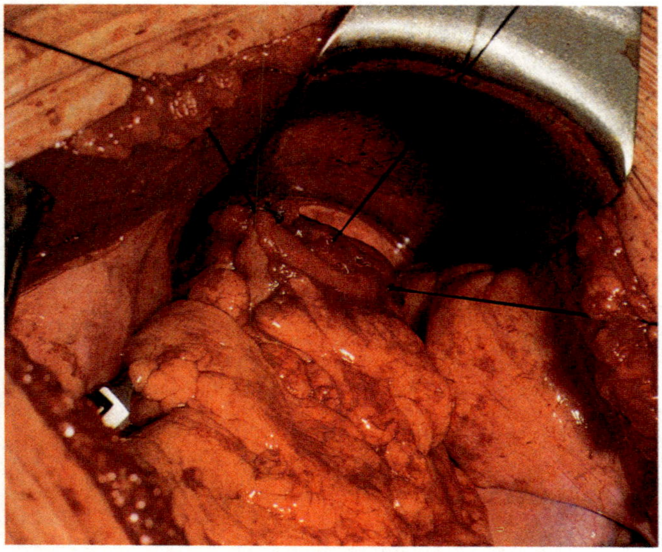

54

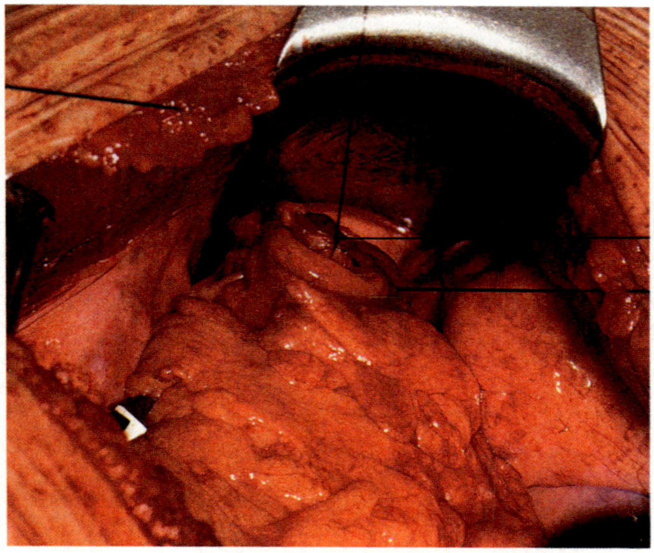

53 The second all-coats Dexon suture is now started, just to the right of the first one near the middle of the posterior wall. Stitching then proceeds to the right along the posterior wall, the right corner is turned, and the suture is 'locked' and turned into a Connell stitch for the front wall. The two sutures are continued, from left to right and from right to left, along the anterior wall, and are tied together in the middle, thus inverting all the anterior wall.

54 The Dexon stitches have been completed, the anterior wall is inverted and the two sutures have been cut. The two end silk stitches are still held.

55 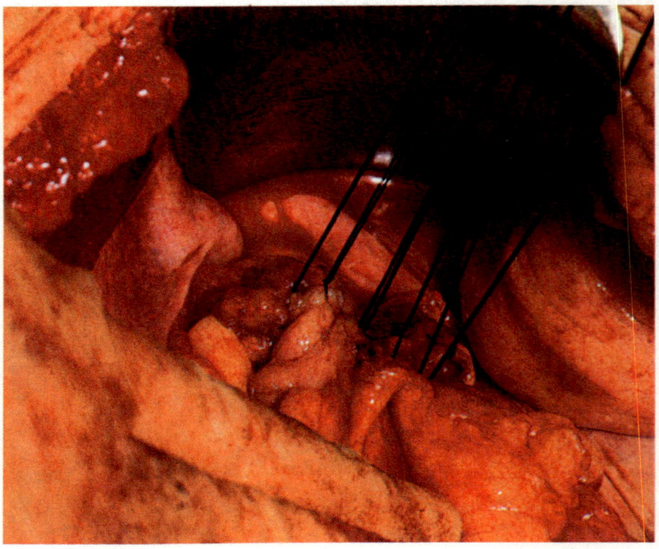

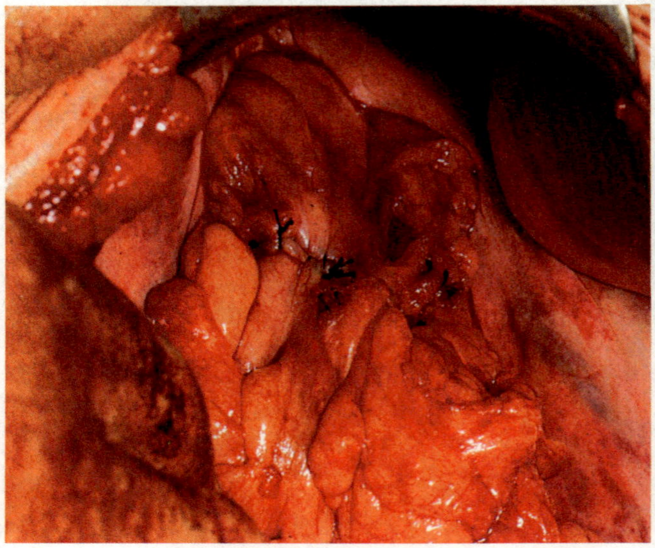 56

55 A few seromuscular stitches are placed along the front wall, further inverting and reinforcing it.

56 The anastomosis is now complete. All stitches are now cut.

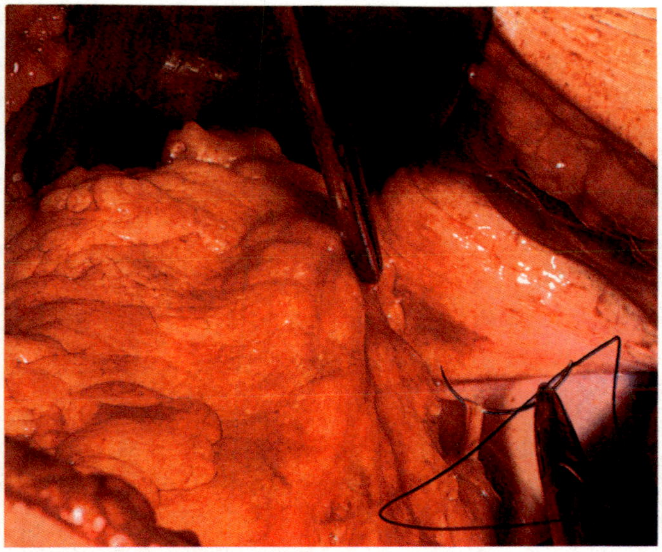

57 The pelvic floor is now closed on the right side. A continuous atraumatic catgut stitch can be used, or interrupted silk as shown here. Stitching starts just above the anastomosis, sewing the right cut edge of peritoneum to the fat or peritoneum of the mesocolon.

Stitching is continued up to the point of ligature of the superior haemorrhoidal vessels, and buries that ligature.

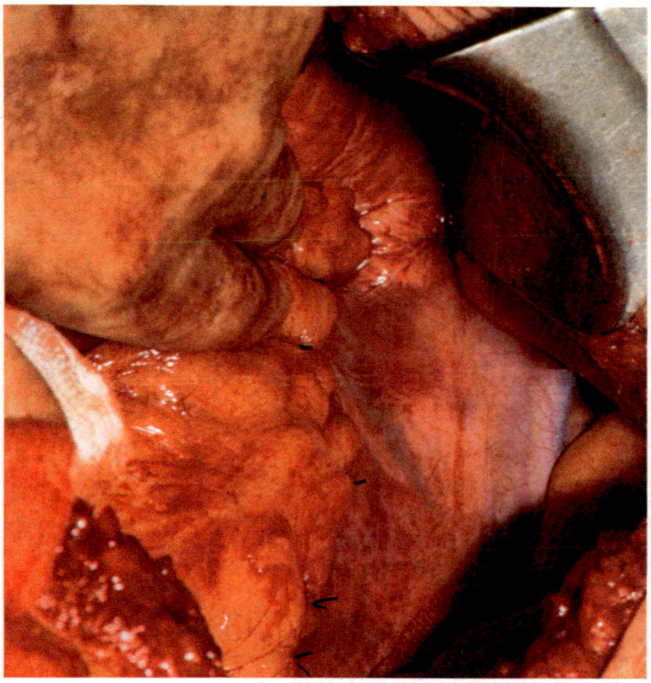

58 The right pelvic floor is now closed.

59

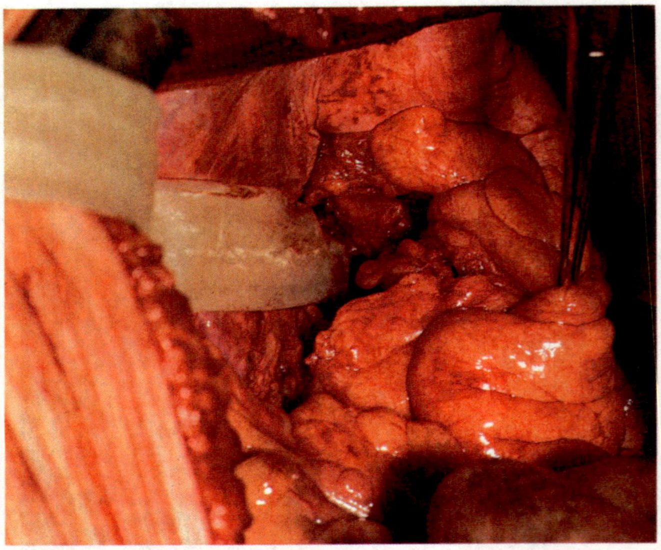

59 On the left side a drain is placed into the hollow of the sacrum, behind the anastomosis, and brought out later through a stab incision in the left iliac fossa. Shown here is a corrugated drain inside a soft tube but other drains, with or without suction, may be used according to preference.

60

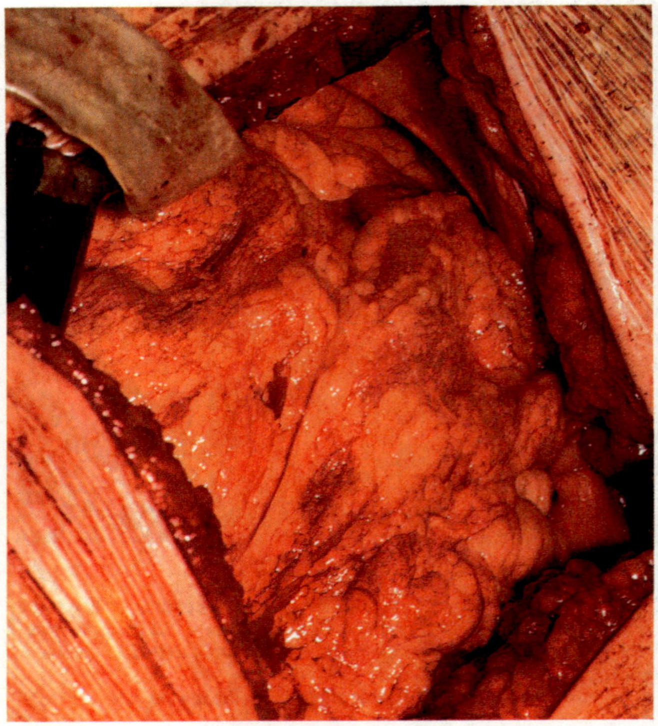

60 Before making the stab for the drain, the omentum should, if possible, be brought down to the pelvis to cover the drain.

The pack holding back the small bowel is then removed and the abdomen closed.

Low and ultra-low anterior resection with stapled anastomosis

Principles

Much of the technique is similar to that which has already been illustrated. The Lloyd-Davies position (Figures 1–4) facilitates both insertion of the gun in favourable cases and the performance of abdomino-perineal excision if this should prove necessary. The incision for the 'low' case should usually extend from xiphisternum to pubis to facilitate mobilisation of the splenic flexure above and the difficult pelvic dissection below.

The early steps of the operation are as already described (Figures **5–9**, pages 11–13).

61

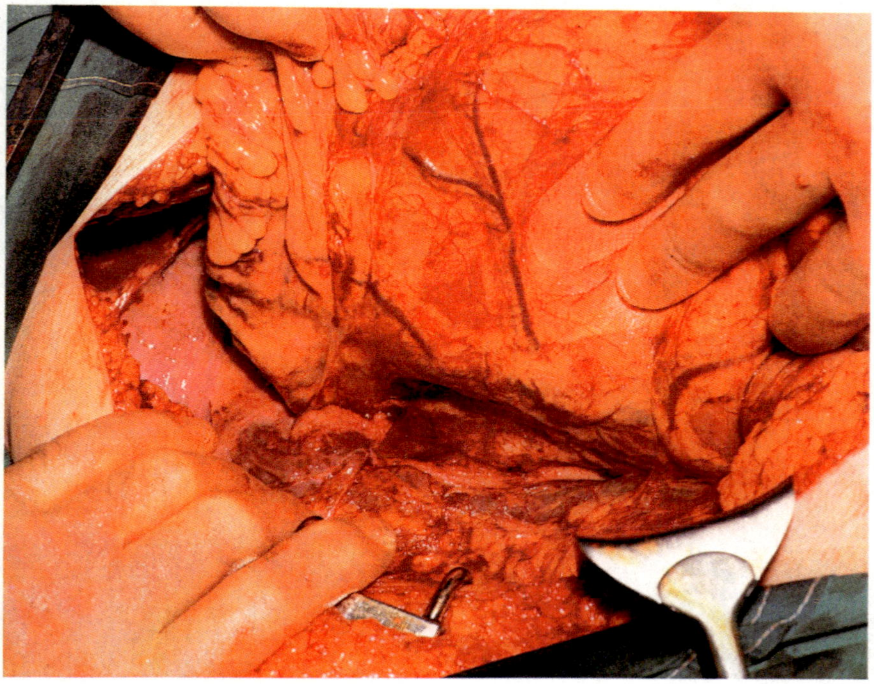

61 The left colon, lifted upwards and to the right by the assistant, is carefully dissected off the posterior abdominal wall preserving ureter, gonadal vessels, and autonomic plexuses.

62

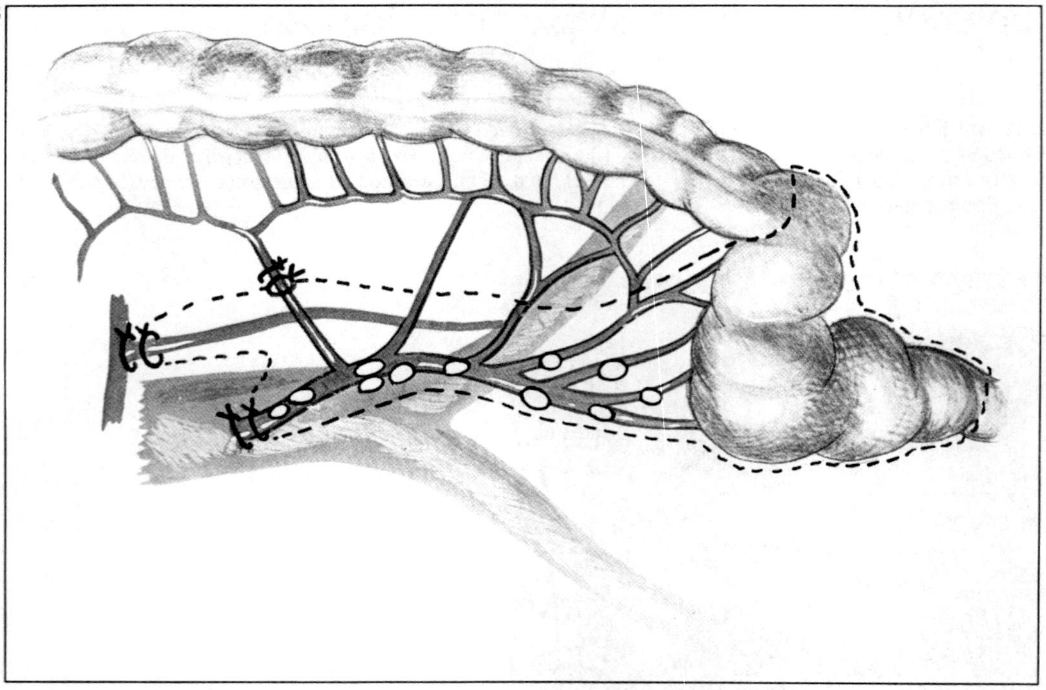

62 In most patients high ligations are necessary to provide sufficient mobility of the left colon for it to reach safely to the pelvic floor.

63

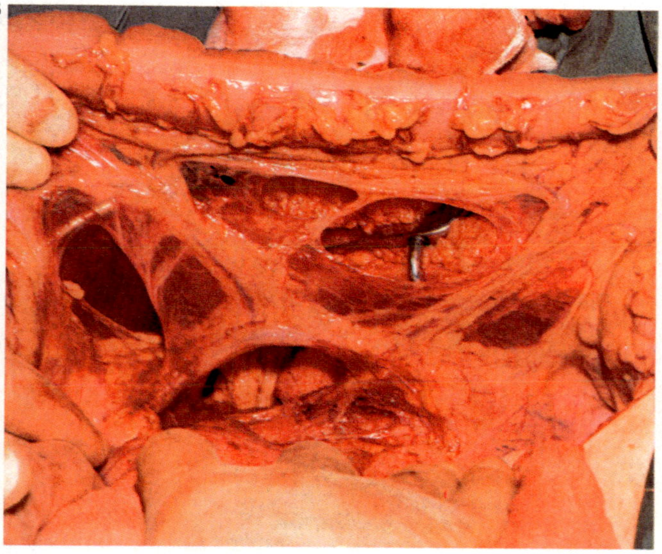

63 (Camera on patient's right side)
The origins of the inferior mesenteric artery from the aorta and of the vein from the splenic vein are identified . . .

64

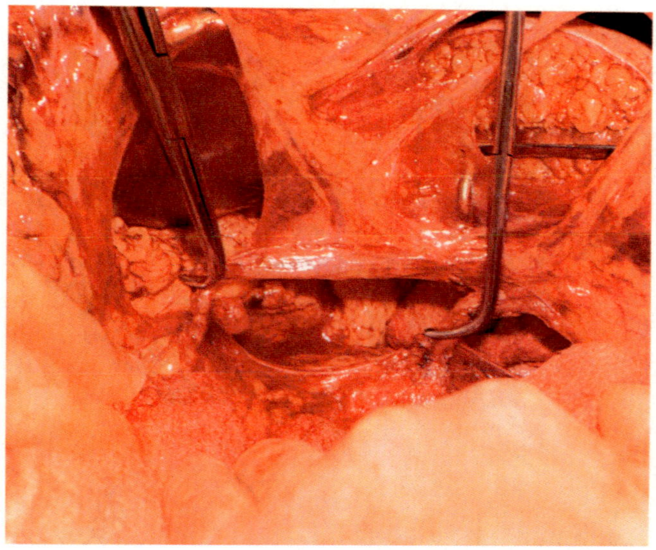

64 . . . and clamped. It is usually possible to preserve the autonomic nerve plexuses which split around the origin of the artery whilst incorporating most nodes in the 'monobloc'.

65 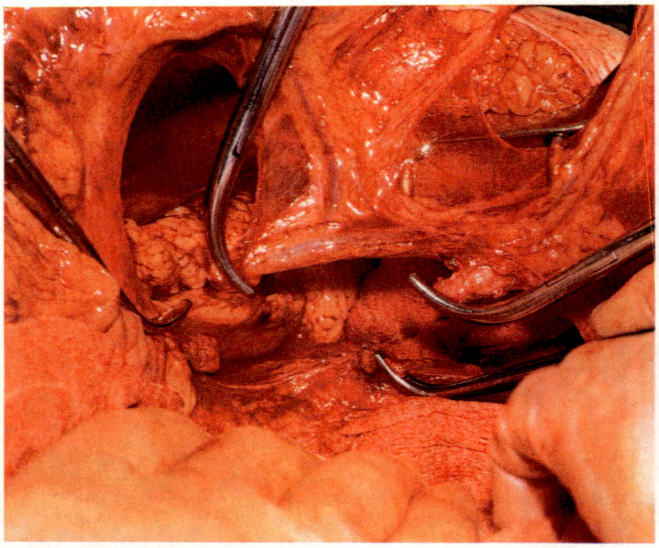

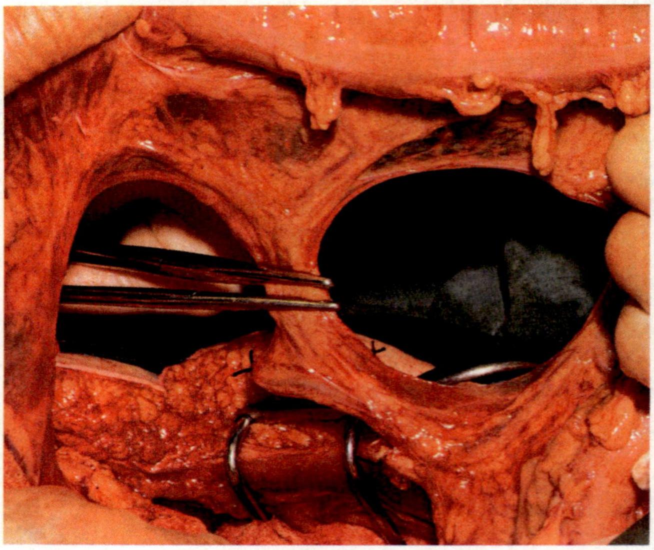 66

65 The vessels are then divided between clamps.
The vein can be taken separately high up if desired: several cm of extra mobility is achieved in this way.

66 The ascending branches of the left colic vessels are divided so as to leave the marginal artery and its arcades intact.

67

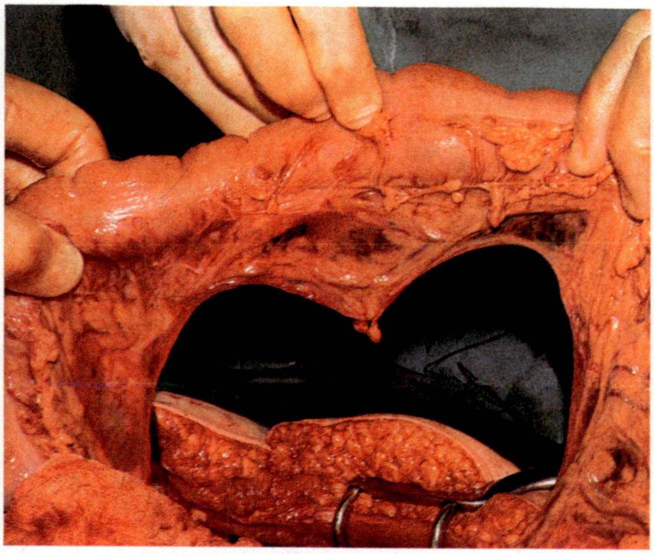

67 Further mobility has been obtained by these vascular divisions and by dissecting the colon away from the left half of the greater omentum.

68

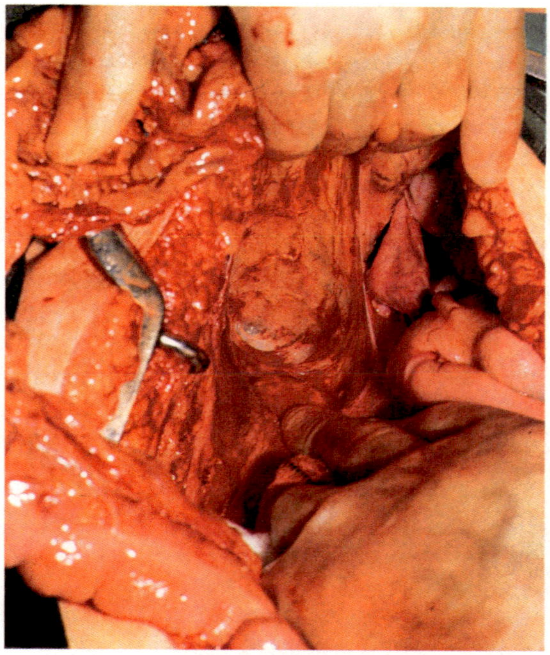

68 Camera now directed into pelvis (rectum held forward)
The most important part of the whole operation is the precise dissection of the rectum and mesorectum (including the whole tumour) out of the pelvis. The clue to the correct plane is the white areolar tissue seen behind the mesorectum in this picture.

69 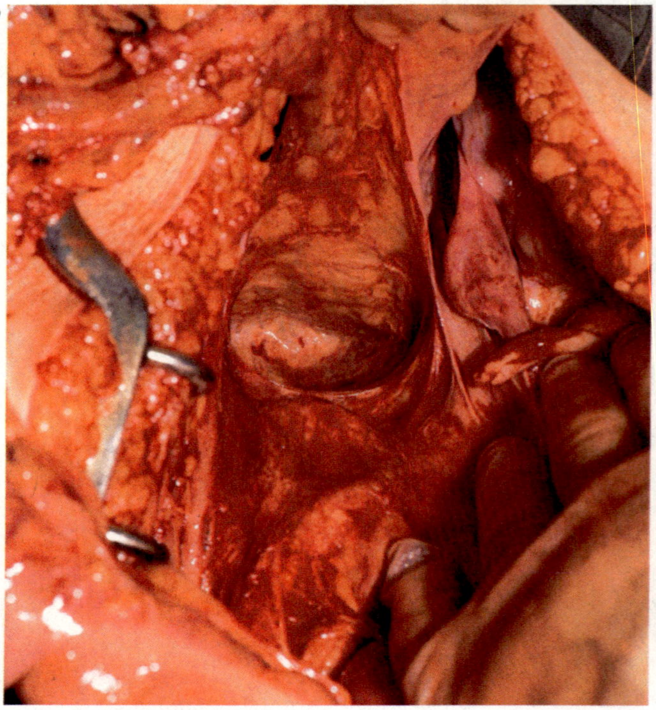 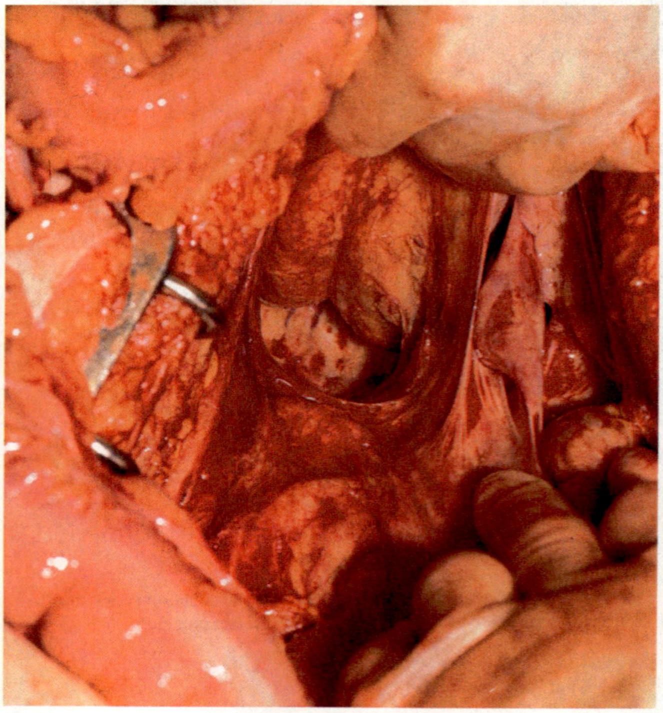 70

69 The best technique is to use sharp scissor dissection under direct vision following the avascular plane within the nerve plexuses. Rarely the tumour seems to transgress this plane and a wider clearance seems necessary.

70 The plane behind the mesorectum is followed right down to the ano-rectal ring. The lowest part of the mesorectum is drawn up with a swab so as to encompass as much of the perirectal lymphatics as possible.

71

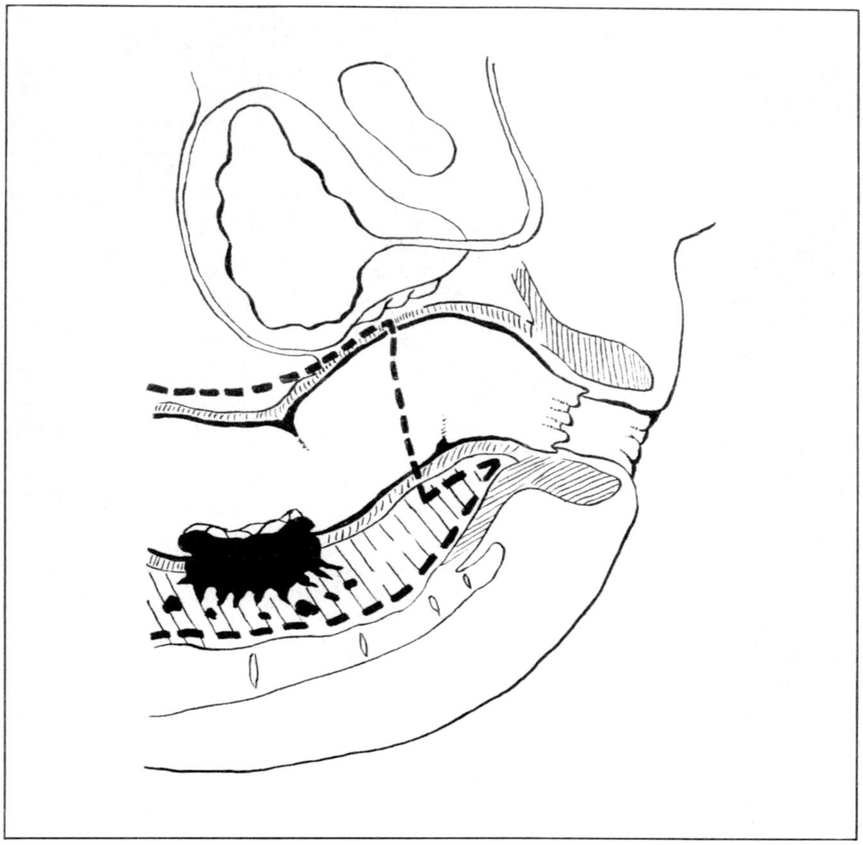

71 Importance is attached to removal of the whole mesorectum so as to empty the pelvis completely of lymphatics close to the tumour.

72

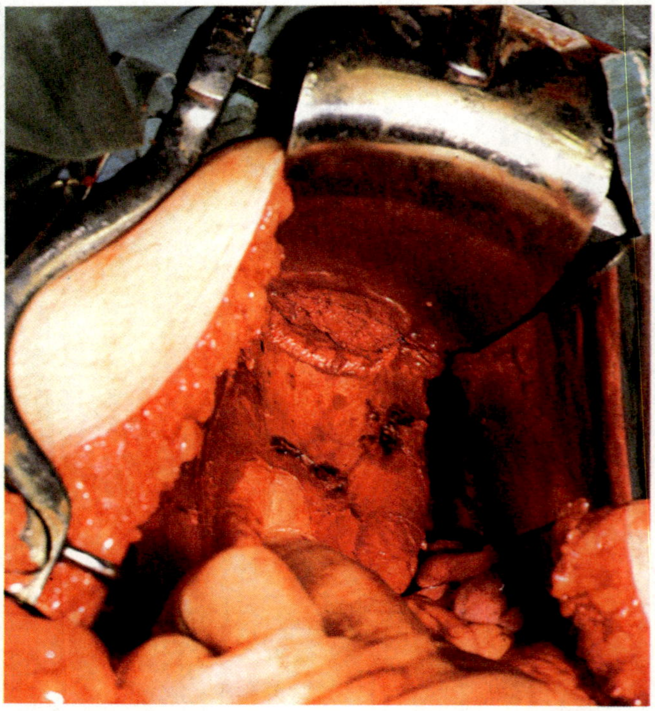

72 The anterior plane is different in the two sexes. Denonvillier's fascia intervenes between the vagina (or prostate) and the rectum and should be excised with the tumour when relevant. Here the vagina is being pushed down and peeled off it . . .

73

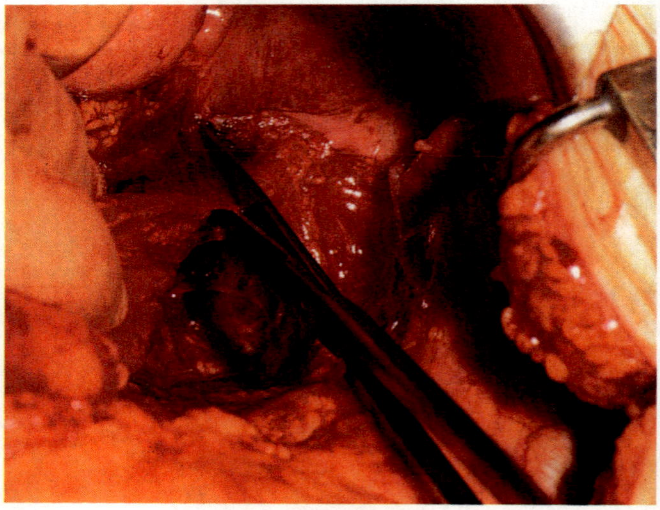

73 When the anterior and posterior dissections have been completed the lateral ligaments or 'stalks' must be divided. Only occasionally does a middle rectal vessel bleed sufficiently to require formal ligation.

74

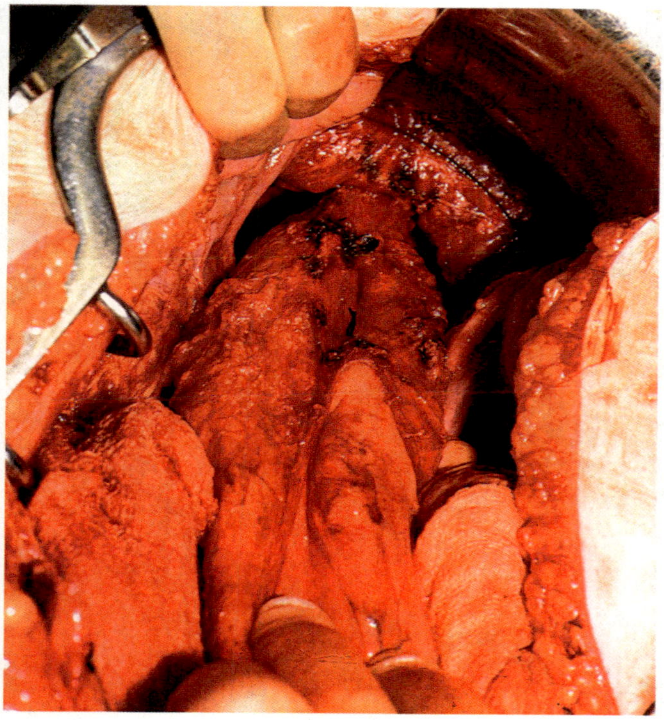

74 The anorectal stump has now been cleared completely of surrounding tissue.

75

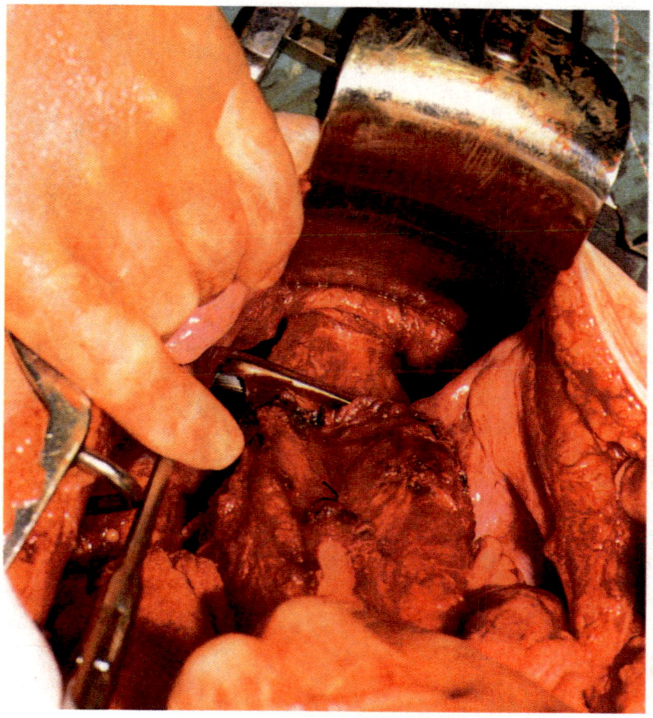

75 It is now cross-clamped with a right-angled clamp. It is sometimes desirable to apply a second clamp in the opposite direction to guard against spillage. At this stage the lower end is washed out with water or with a suitable cytotoxic solution (see Figure **30**).

76

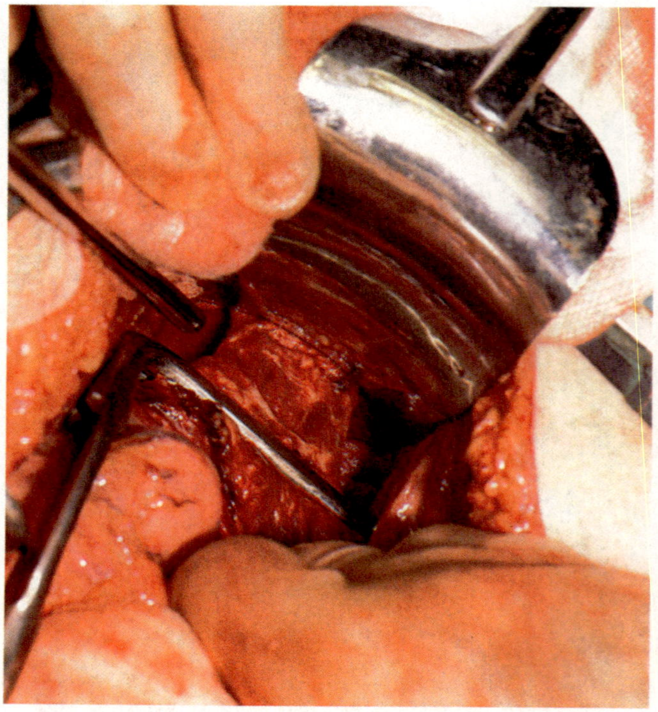

77

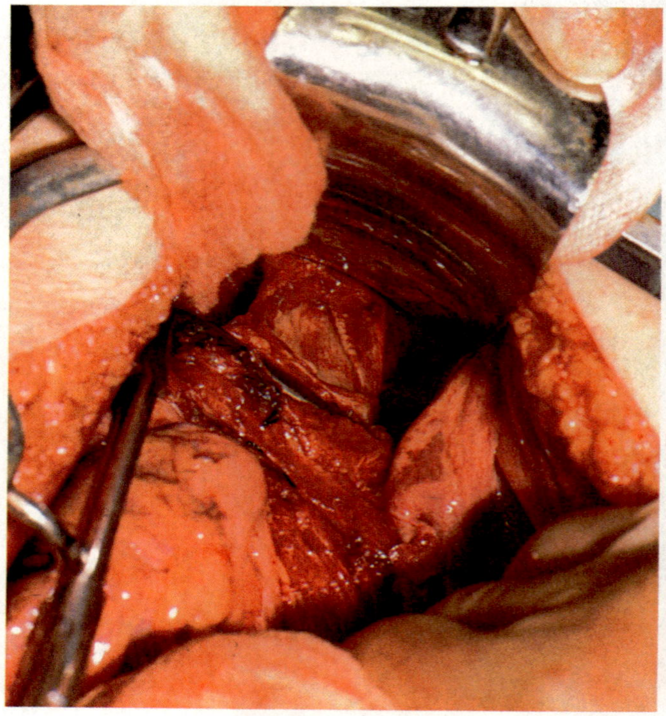

76 Downward traction with the St Mark's retractor and upward traction on the right angled clamp provide access to the lowest part of the anterior wall of the rectum. The muscle layer of the anterior wall is incised with a knife . . .

77 . . . and the mucosa with scissors. The lumen should be clean after the wash-out.

78

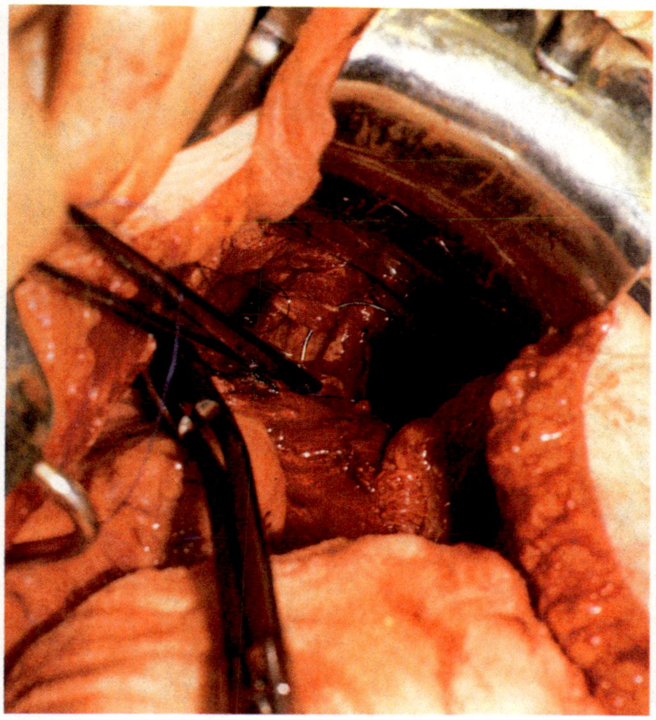

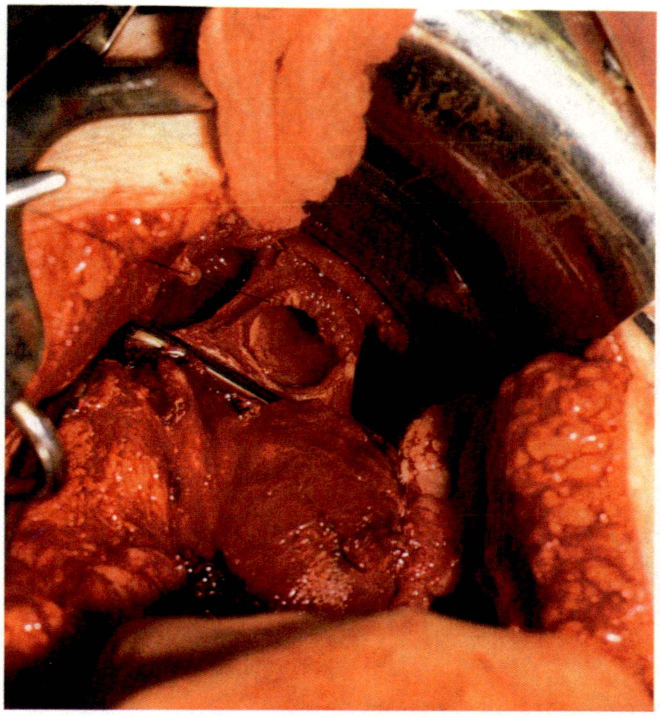

79

78 The purse-string stitch is inserted anteriorly whilst this distortion of the anatomy is maintained. 0 prolene is ideal and an 'over and over' stitch is satisfactory. This should incorporate the mucosa and 2 mm of muscularis mucosae (visible as a thin white line) and the bites should be 5 mm apart.

79 After the anterior wall has been 'purse-stringed' the posterior wall can be cut . . .

80 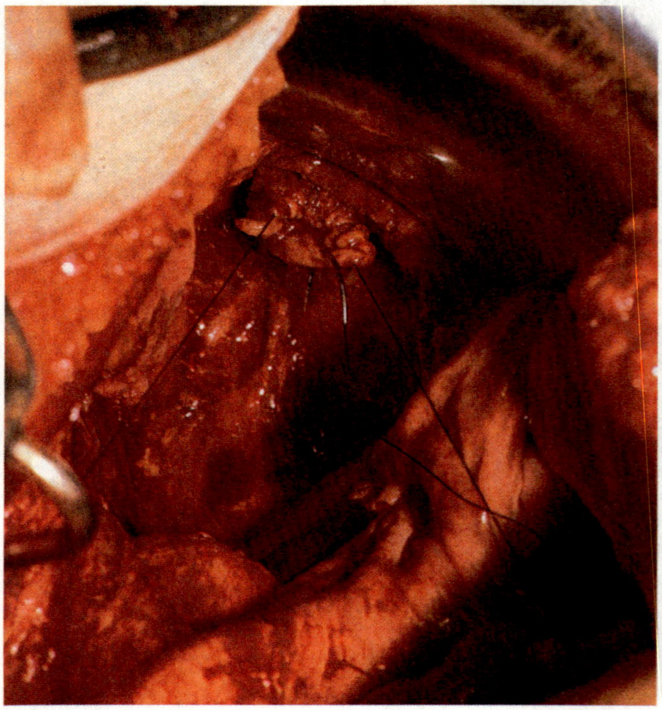

81 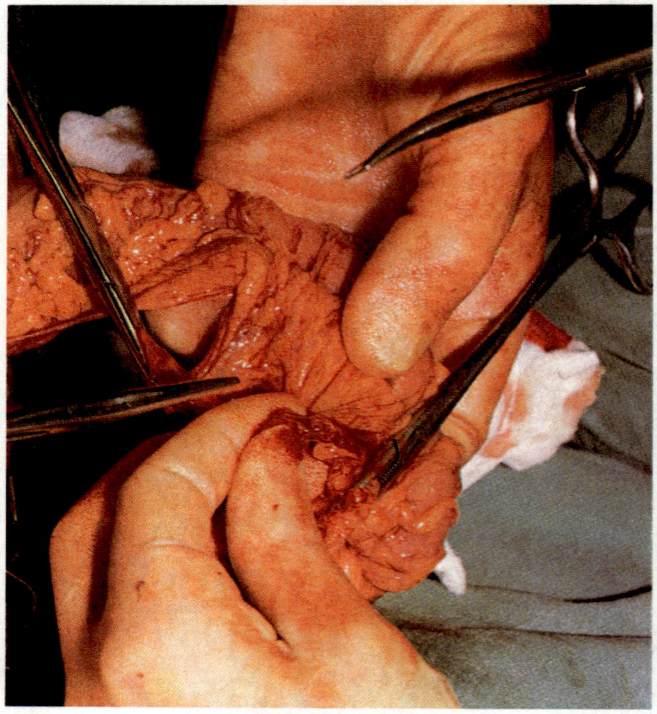

80 . . . and the over and over stitch continued to complete the circle.

81 For the colonic side the blood vessels are divided distal to the intended point of section of the colon.

82

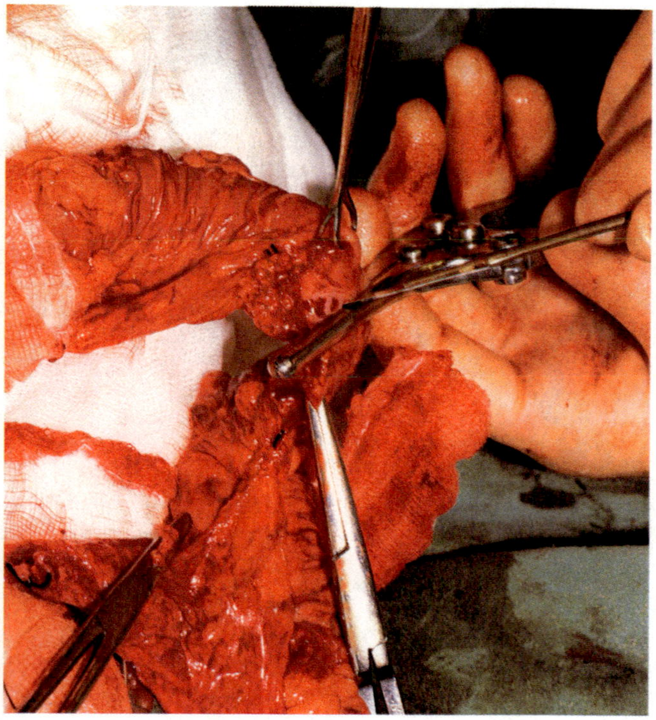

83

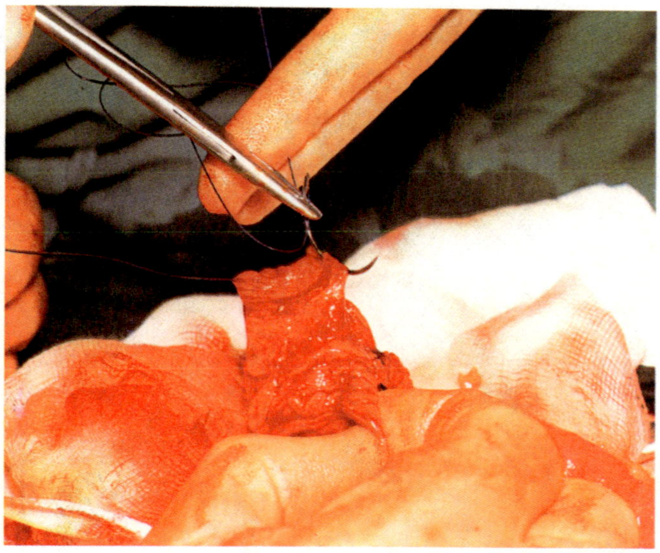

83 The colonic side is now similarly 'purse-stringed' in preparation for 'loading' into the gun.

82 The colon is divided and any residual faecal material sucked out.

84

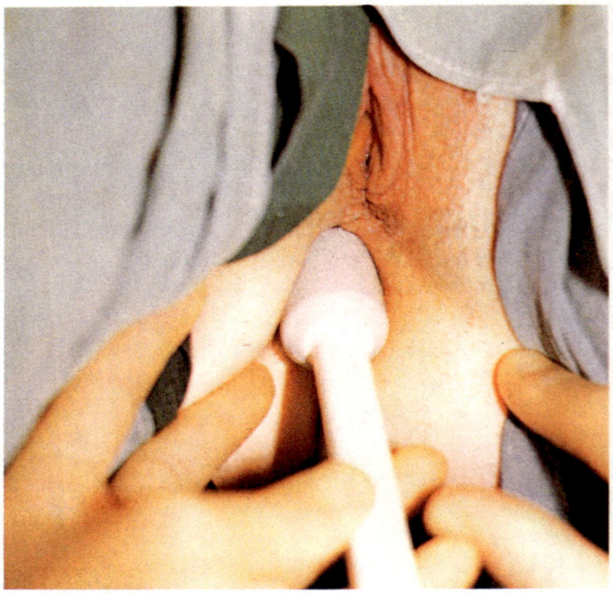

85

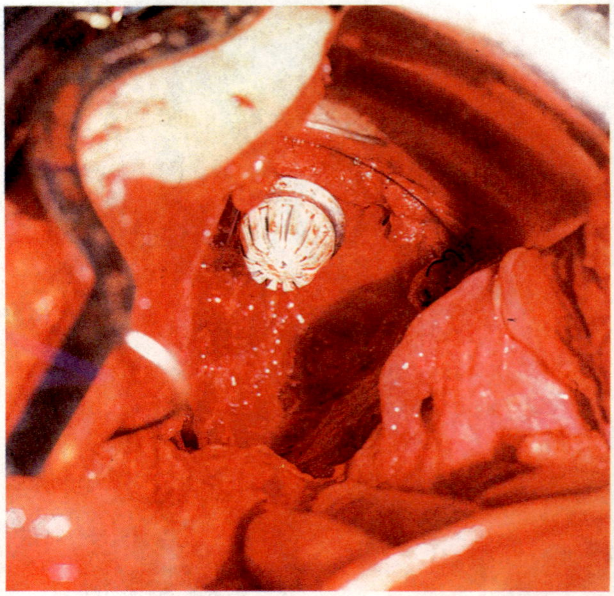

84 and 85 The 'gun' is now inserted by a skilled assistant into the anus and through the anus and rectal stump to appear at the bottom of the pelvis.

86

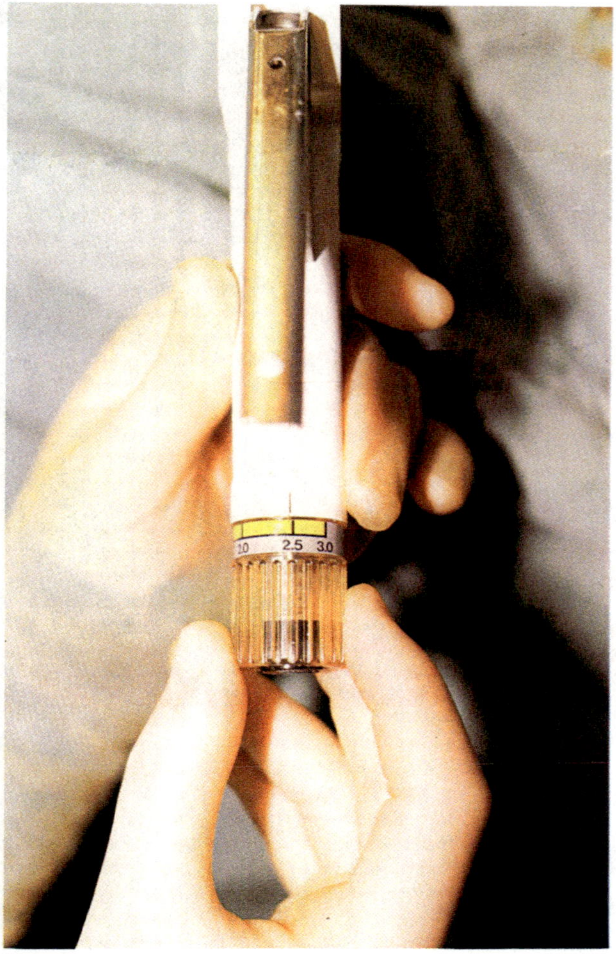

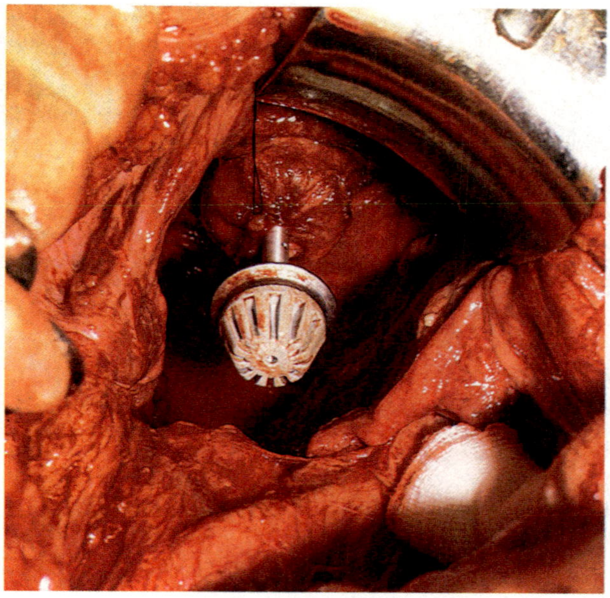

87

86 The gap is opened by unscrewing the gun . . .

87 . . . and the rectal purse-string is tightened firmly down on to the shaft.

88

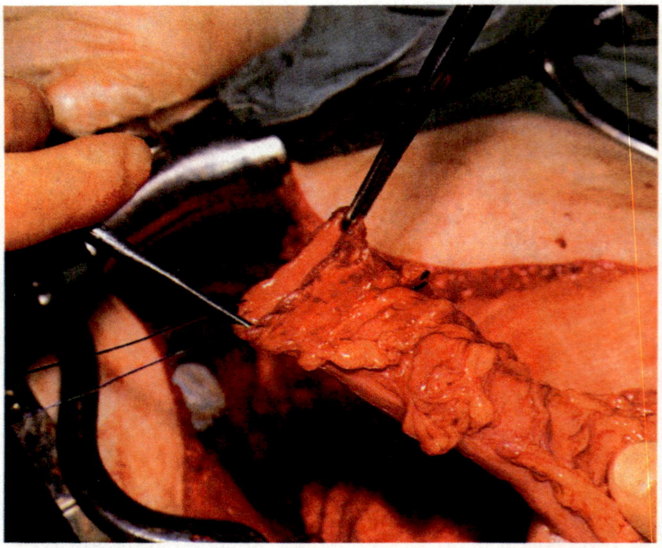

89

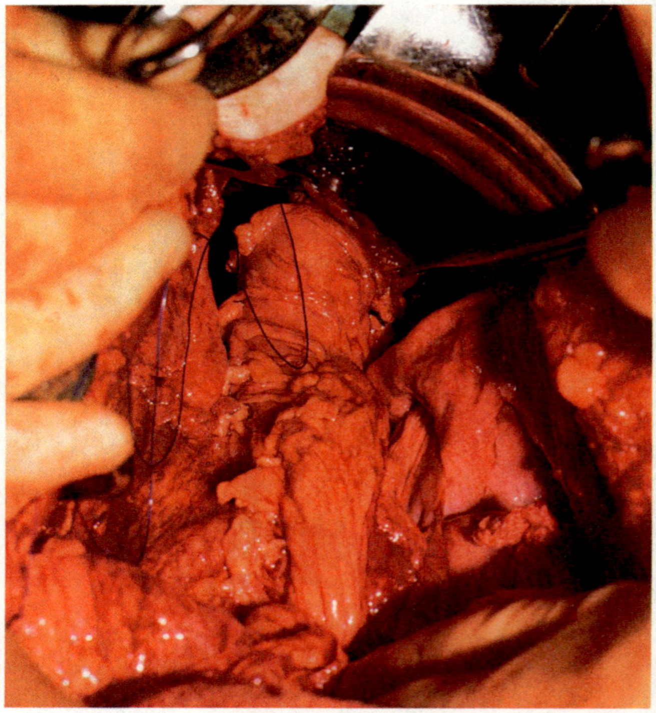

88 The colonic end is ready for the anastomosis and the purse-string is loose.

89 Alliss forceps are used to slip the colonic end over the anvil. The 'saucer' shape of the anvil can be used to do this obliquely.

90

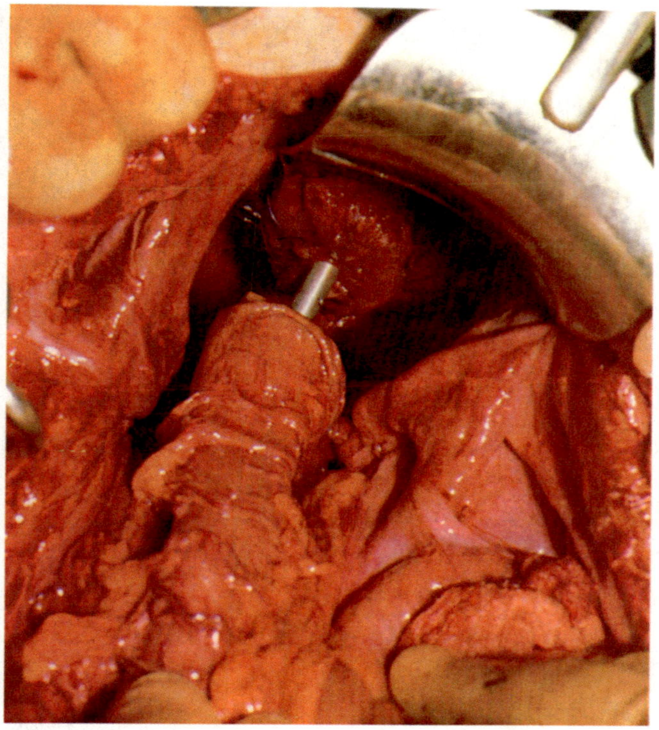

91

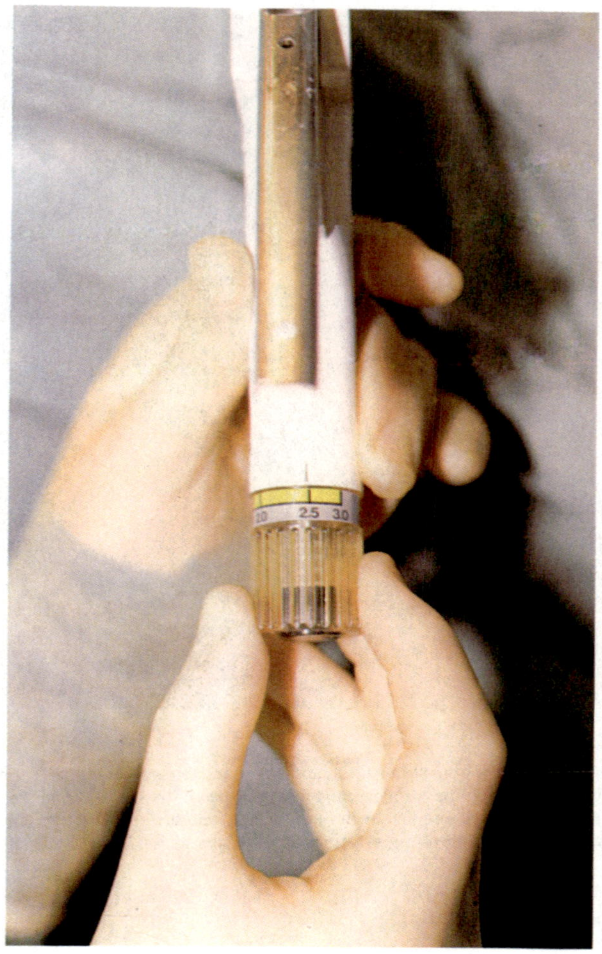

90 The upper purse-string has now also been tied firmly on to the shaft. Care is taken to prevent other tissues from becoming interposed between the ends.

91 The gap is gently closed to around 2–2.5 mm according to the estimated thickness of the 'turn-in'. This is effected by turning the screw on the base of the gun.

92

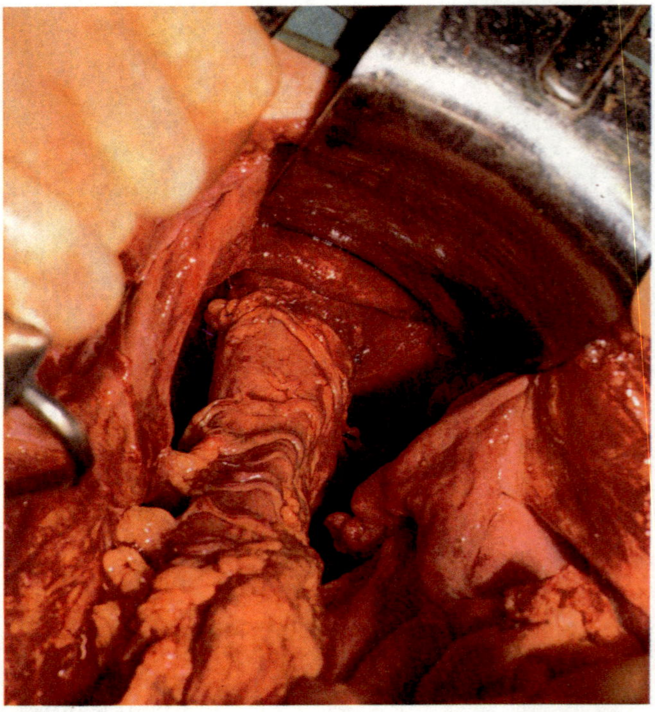

93

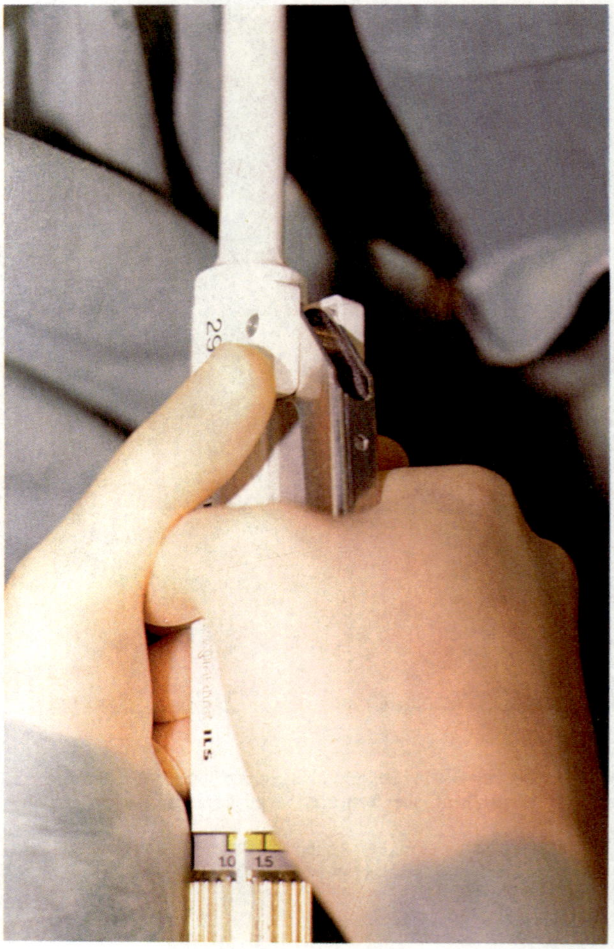

92 and 93 Seen from within the abdomen the ends are now together. The gun is 'fired' by pulling the trigger firmly after release of the safety catch. It is then steadied from above whilst the gun is unscrewed one turn to open the gap and then withdrawn by gentle tilting, traction and possibly rotation.

4
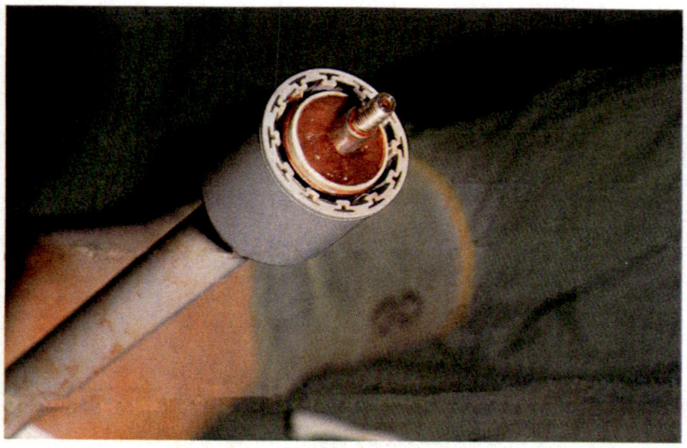

5
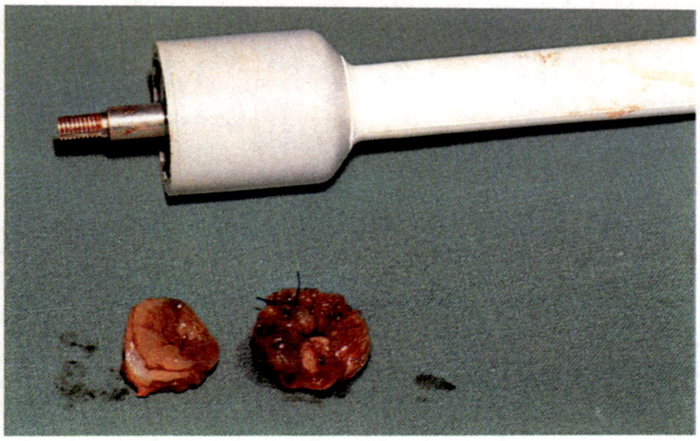

96
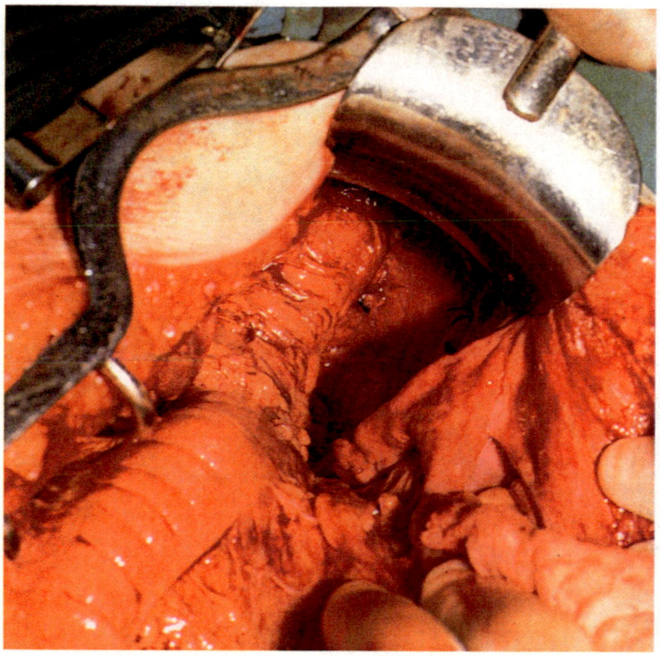

94 When the anvil is unscrewed the so-called 'doughnuts' of bowel ends can be seen within the head of the 'gun'.

95 It is important that a complete circle of tissue should be present in each. If either is incomplete the anastomosis will be eccentric and a defect will probably be present.

96 The colon should lie without tension in the hollow of the pelvis. It is essential that it should *not* be stretched across the front of the pelvis with a residual cavity posteriorly.

97 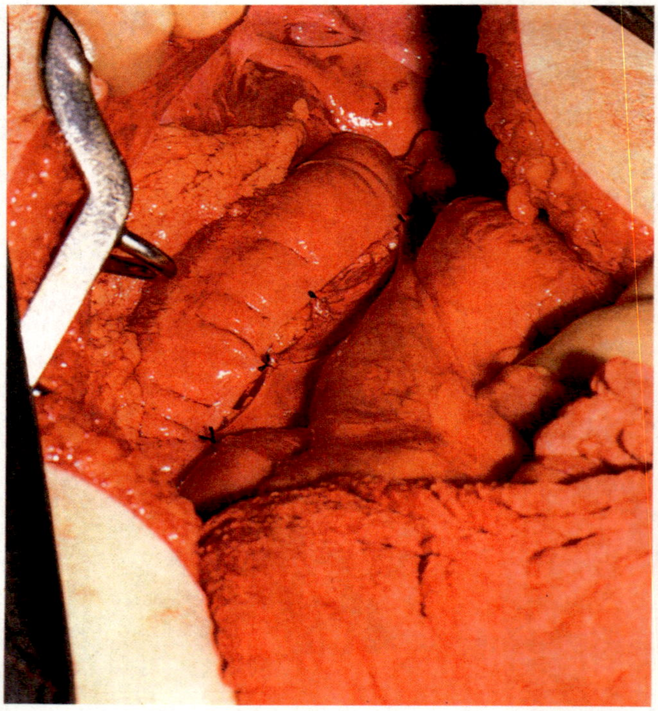

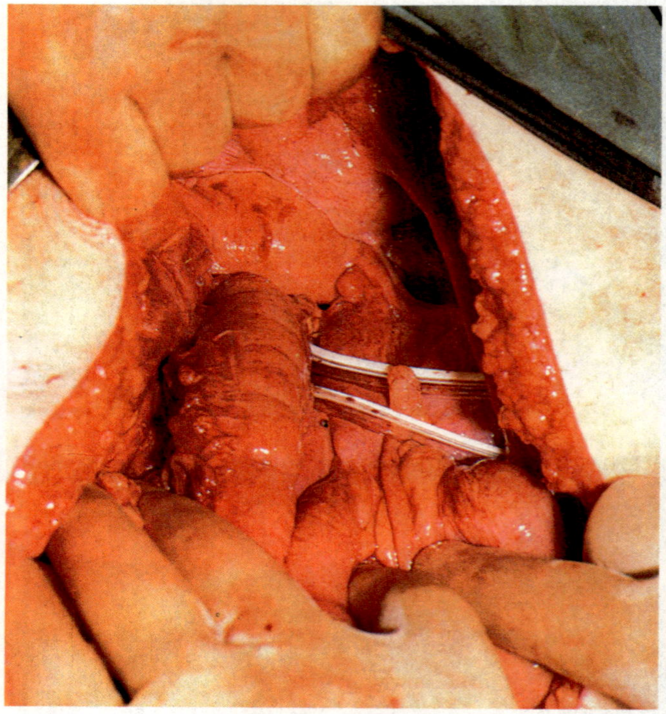 98

97 Pelvic 'filling' with redundant bowel and/or with the mobilised greater omentum is desirable. Even the caecum can be mobilised and used for this purpose if necessary. A few stitches have been added on the right side to prevent retro-colic herniation.

98 Drainage of the extensively emptied and dissected pelvis is essential since residual haematoma and sero-sanguinous collections will become infected and may cause a 'late leak'. Two suction pump drains have been used here. A Penrose drain as illustrated earlier is an alternative.

99

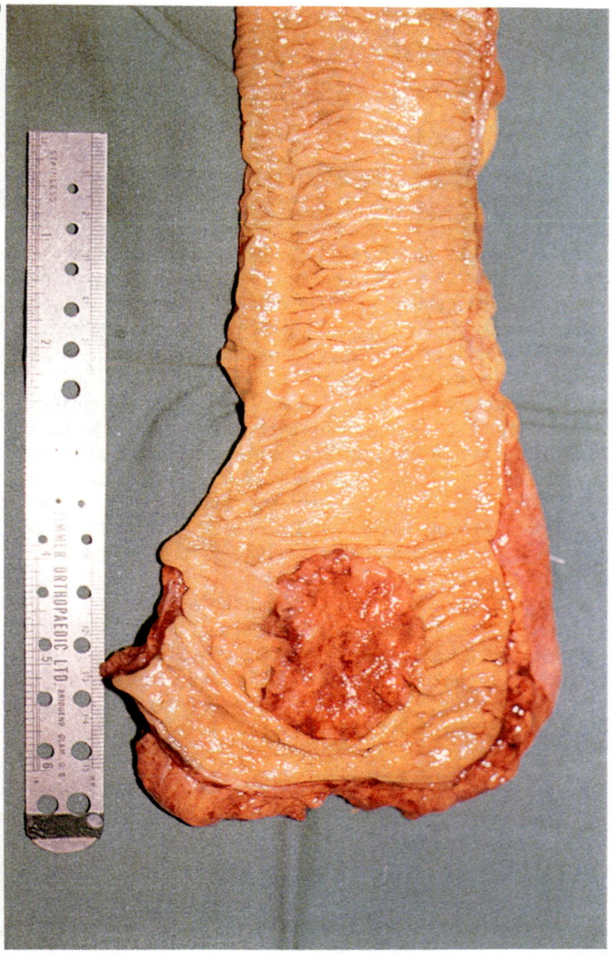

99 If the tumour is poorly differentiated or the distal margin considered less than adequate (2 cm or less) then immediate frozen section examination of the distal edge is desirable. The operation should be converted to a total excision if the tissue is found to be invaded, though this is rare in the common differentiated type of lesion.

Is a transverse colostomy necessary?

The authors' preference is for 4–6 weeks protection by a transverse loop colostomy in all 'ultra-low' anastomoses, i.e. those within 6–7 cm of the anal verge. For higher anastomoses this precaution can reasonably be omitted provided that every aspect of the surgery has been satisfactory. Properly executed and carefully closed, a transverse colostomy should produce few extra problems and is always a wise precaution if there is any doubt. Furthermore, in the ultra-low case, the patient will often experience transitory problems of rectal frequency and urgency in the first few weeks and these are more easily borne when he or she has fully recovered from the main operation.

Variations in the operation according to the extent of the tumour

It has already been suggested that the 5 cm mural clearance may be reduced to 2 cm in differentiated lesions but that the whole *mesorectum* (or at least 5 cm of it) should be incorporated to provide wide perirectal lymphatic clearance in every case. The proximal extent of the resection is probably less important. Thus a 'flush tie' with lymphatic clearance up to the inferior mesenteric origin confers only marginal advantages in terms of tumour clearance – but in an elderly person undergoing high anterior resection it would add significantly to the magnitude and risk of the procedure. For the low anterior resection high division of the vessels is necessary for mobilisation and only secondarily for the added lymphatic clearance.

Adherence of other organs should not be regarded with inordinate gloom. In more than half of those cases where small bowel, bladder, or uterus are adherent to the primary the subsequent histology reveals no evidence of actual tumour invasion: i.e. the adherence is due to inflammation and does not significantly affect prognosis. Indeed size and even direct invasion of other tissues worsen the outlook much less than the discovery of the smallest distant metastasis.

The pre-operative IVP may help the surgeon to decide whether an involved ureter should be locally removed and tied off as the kidney is non-functional, or an attempt made to reimplant it if it is visualised below a functional kidney. If both kidneys are functioning one ureter may be tied off in the reasonable expectation that the kidney will atrophy. Nephrectomy is perhaps to be preferred if it does not add too much to the magnitude of the operation.

The vaginal vault is a well recognised site for recurrent disease. The need to excise its posterior wall because of an anterior growth usually but not invariably implies an abdomino-perineal excision. Sometimes however the sphincter can be preserved and a low anastomosis performed despite an extensive clearance which includes the uterus and the upper two thirds of the posterior vaginal wall. In such cases the undoubted risk of recto-vaginal fistula can be reduced by interposition of the mobilised omentum plus protection by a defunctioning colostomy.

Certain large tumours seem to demand a wider lateral clearance incorporating the endo-pelvic fascia and even the internal iliac vessels on one side. Straying laterally in the pelvis from the 'natural' avascular plane does, however, involve a risk of increased blood loss as well as a virtual certainty of impotence and an anaesthetic bladder. More extensive lymphadenectomy around the origin of the inferior mesenteric artery or even along the pelvic brim may occasionally seem relevant and confers less in the way of neurological defect.

Occasionally an anterior tumour in a male invades the back of the bladder. In such cases, if local removal of a disc of bladder apparently clears the malignant disease, anterior resection may still be appropriate. Omentum should be interposed between the bladder suture line and the anastomosis at the end of the operation and the catheter in the bladder should be retained for ten days.

Distant metastasis (Figure 100)

In most patients who are found at laparotomy to have hepatic metastases, the removal of the primary tumour by anterior resection should proceed as planned. This will prevent distressing symptoms and perhaps obstruction due to the primary tumour. In only a few cases with massive involvement of the liver or widespread peritoneal metastasis should resection of the primary be abandoned.

A *solitary* hepatic metastasis does provide the surgeon with a particular challenge. Segmentectomy, hemi-hepatectomy or local excision, either immediate or delayed, offer the patient his only chance of permanent cure. Assessment for hepatic resection should ideally include a CAT scan and a hepatic arteriogram so that other metastases may be detected and the vascular anatomy defined. Thus delayed hepatic resection after recovery from the initial operation is probably the method of choice in most cases.

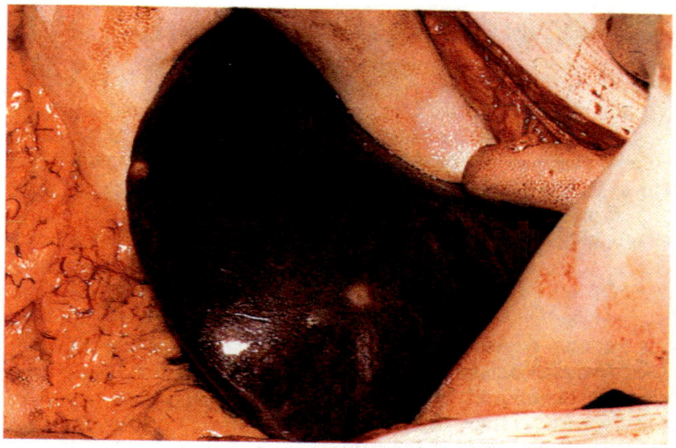

100

Operative problems specific to 'gun anastomoses'

In the early days 'withdrawal' problems were sometimes encountered, i.e. the gun 'fired' but could not readily be withdrawn from the patient. This particularly occurred with the SPTU gun if the washer was worn or distorted such that the knife did not cut cleanly. To a lesser extent it is still inclined to occur with the disposable EEA cartridges because the knife may trap mucosa in the washer without cutting it completely; gentle rotation of the open gun will usually tear this free without disrupting the anastomosis itself. If the gun is firmly impacted the gap should be fully opened and the anastomosis drawn down if possible and cut free under direct vision. This process may be facilitated by insertion of a Parks retractor around the shaft.

The commonest problems are due to unsatisfactory insertion of the lower purse-string. Multiple deep bites of bulky rectal muscle may produce a purse-string which fails to 'run' so that it does not close down on to the spindle. Too few bites may lead to a part of the circumference being squeezed out when the gun is closed. Indeed the proper insertion of the lower purse-string is the essence of 'gun technique'.

The 'incomplete doughnut' may reflect an eccentric anastomosis and a probable defect. It should alert the surgeon to perform a washout which may demonstrate the site of the leak so that an extra suture may be inserted. Such a suspect anastomosis should certainly be protected by a defunctioning colostomy.

Post-operative complications

General principles directed towards avoidance of thrombo-embolic complications are of paramount importance since all major pelvic operations are high-risk cases for venous thrombosis. Indeed mortality is in most series virtually confined to the elderly in whom such problems predominate. The transverse colostomy calls for sympathetic stomatherapy advice and often as much of the stomatherapist's time as the permanent colostomist. The major complication which is specific to anterior resection is anastomotic leakage. The risk of this increases as the distance from the anus diminishes, with 10–20% of colo-anal and low rectal anastomoses reported as 'leaks' in most series. The causes include infected pelvic haematoma and a relative inadequacy of the colonic blood supply amounting rarely to actual necrosis. The consequences vary from an asymptomatic sinus detectable only by x-ray to a dangerous and persistent pelvic sepsis or even spreading peritonitis. A discharge of flatus or a minor faecal leak from the drain can be treated expectantly, but serious leakage in a patient unprotected by proximal colostomy involves urgent exploration and effective defunctioning. This may need to be supplemented by complete emptying of the colon distal to the colostomy by lavage and suction. If a colostomy has already been performed at the time of the operation and this appears to be functioning correctly then expectant treatment will generally suffice. Only rarely will the condition of the patient and the physical signs dictate exploration to exclude bowel necrosis or faecal leakage due to 'spill-over' at the colostomy. Closure of the colostomy in all these cases will have to be deferred until a radio-opaque enema shows that the anastomosis has healed. In some patients a large posterior diverticulum may persist and become epithelialised, and closure may have to wait for 6–12 months.

Another complication which may be seen after anterior resection is small bowel obstruction. In addition to band obstruction, which can occur after any abdominal operation, it may occur after anterior resection when a space has been left behind the bowel in the hollow of the sacrum into which prolapse of ileum occurs during the days after surgery. If the bowel is friable it can be difficult and dangerous to deal with and it is much better to prevent it by filling the pelvis with mobilised and redundant colon plus omentum or caecum if necessary.

The radio-opaque enema

This is essential prior to the closure of an established colostomy and sometimes of value in investigating post-operative complications. A water-soluble medium and *not* barium should be used. It is not, however, without its dangers since the anterior part of a low staple-line is easily disrupted by the careless insertion of a rigid enema nozzle. The x-ray department should therefore be warned of the existence of a low anastomosis so that special care can be taken. Since transverse colostomy closure is probably technically easier after 4–6 weeks there is an argument for delaying the enema for 3–4 weeks after surgery when healing will be more secure. A straight x-ray is of some value since an intact ring of staples after several weeks usually indicates a properly healed anastomosis (Figure **101**). Where leakage has occurred the usual x-ray finding is of a posterior cavity communicating with the lumen through or just above the ring of staples (Figure **102**).

101a

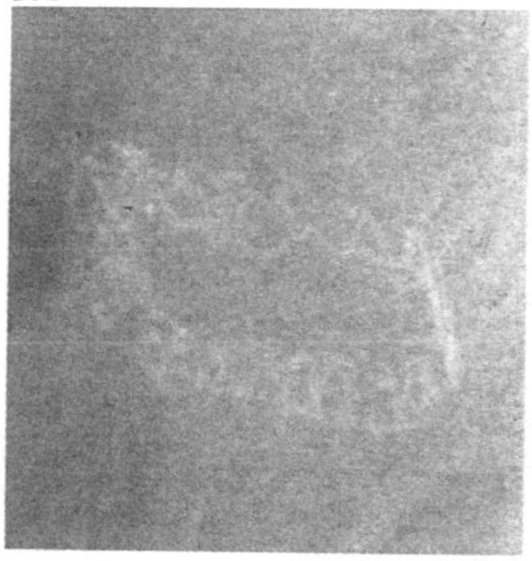

101b

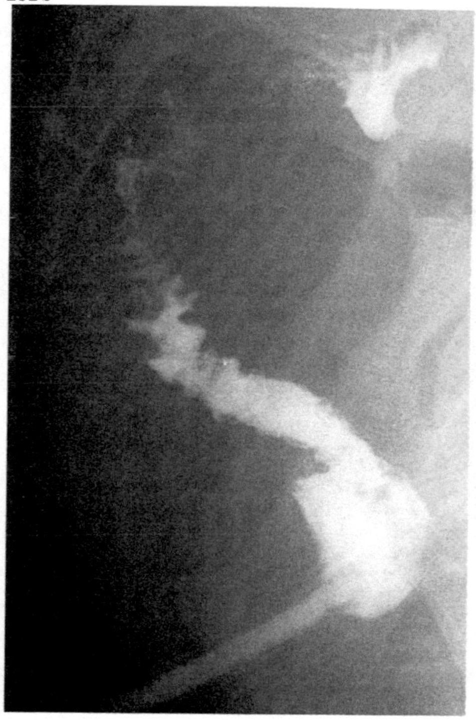

101c

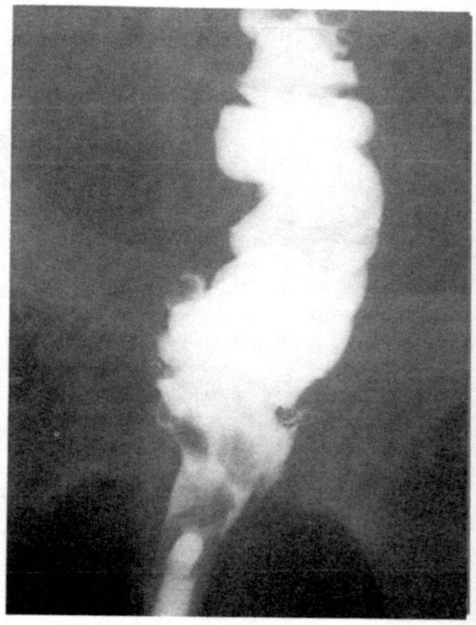

101a-c An intact ring of staples on a straight x-ray (**101a**) usually indicates an intact anastomosis on the gastrografin enema (**101b** and **101c**).

102

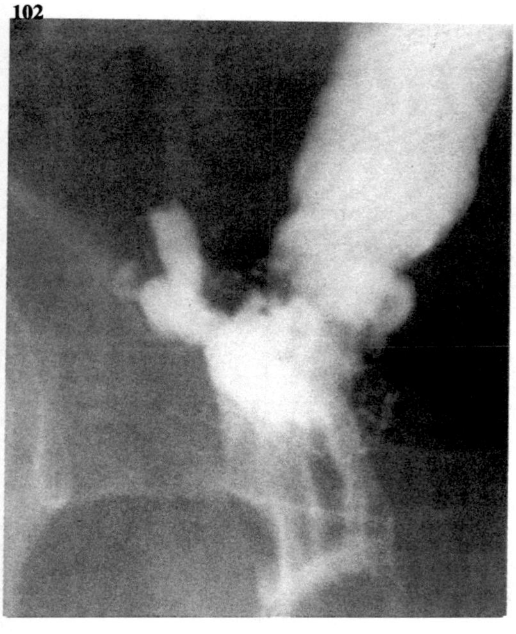

Index

FSC
www.fsc.org
MIX
Papier | Fördert gute Waldnutzung
FSC® C083411

Zeitfracht Medien GmbH
Ferdinand-Jühlke-Straße 7
99095 Erfurt, Deutschland
produktsicherheit@kolibri360.de